Plant-Based

WELL KIND OF

Cookbook

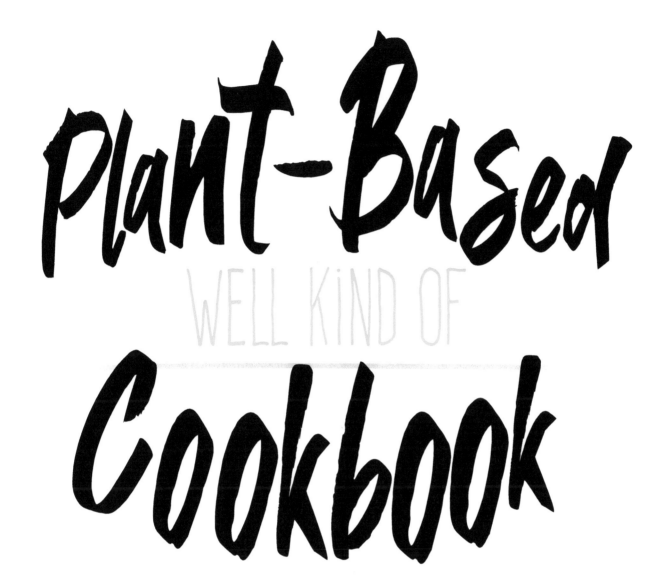

Plant-Based

WELL KIND OF

Cookbook

CALIE CALABRESE AND NIC HEFFERNAN

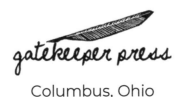

gatekeeper press

Columbus, Ohio

Plant-Based Cookbook: Well Kind Of

Published by Gatekeeper Press
2167 Stringtown Rd, Suite 109
Columbus, OH 43123-2989
www.GatekeeperPress.com

The cover design, and editorial work for this book are entirely the product
of the author. Gatekeeper Press did not participate in and is not responsible
for any aspect of these elements.

ISBN (hardcover): 9781662900068

CALIE'S DEDICATION

To all of the guardian angels sent to guide me on my journey throughout the years. Those named and those whose names I've forgotten but whose acts of kindness I never will.

Sarah F & Jenny McG...you two and your families were my saving grace in high school. People tell me all the time I should be dead or a drug addict and I honestly think it was having friends like you guys and the way your families took me in and showed me love and caring during some of the most challenging times that kept me on a positive path. There's not enough room in this book for all of our stories or all of my thanks, but I love you guys!

To my college roommate, Michelle, and her family for the gift of a family Christmas my freshman year. You'll never know how much that experience meant to me.

To the family in Chicago that gave me a home and trusted me with your kids, while I completed my internship. Thank you!

To Jen, Amelia, Lindsay, Mere and Kendra...thank you for your friendship, your texts, your visits, our wine nights and all of the millions of little ways you helped the boys and I through the divorce. I'm so grateful for your friendship!

To my sister, Autumn, for taking me and the boys in when we had nothing and for giving me the opportunity to participate in *80 Day Obsession* where I found mental strength while building physical strength. I love you!

And to Nic, for embracing my crazy idea to write a cookbook together and stepping way outside of his comfort zone to make it a reality. Thank you for your creativity, making me laugh, keeping me grounded, and calling me out on my bullshit. I'm glad we were both dickheads 3 years ago so that we could lose our way and end up on our journeys. Journeys that taught us the lessons we needed to transform into the people we are today. I love you!

NIC'S DEDICATION

To my best mate Wai. You are one of the hardest workers I have ever met. You have been working since the age of 12, striving to be a more educated, more of a rounded person. I learnt so much from you and continue to do so. What an amazing person to have in my corner.

To my best mates Ricky and Brianna. Thank you for being honest and direct with me at my low points. You will always be the person people look up to for guidance and will always come out a better person from meeting you. Brianna, you are a hilarious, loving and caring person who has been through more than most, but you continue to have the strength to keep being. I'm so proud of you.

To my long childhood friend Tom. You have had a hard go at it, especially in your younger days. It could have been easy for you to go down a dark path. But you stuck at it, are happily married and one of the most humble and caring men I have ever met. I have known you since I was 5 and consider myself lucky to have you in my life all these years later.

To my Mum, Eric and Sisters. Mum, thank you for raising me the way you did. You are hilarious and have such an incredible sense of humor. Thank you for sticking with me and continuing to show your love and support. Eric, what a hard worker and good man. Thank you for making my mum happy with your ridiculous humor. You make us all laugh! Kerrie and Jodie, I hope someday we can reconnect. I look back at our childhood and it was amazing! We were three peas in a pod.

To David and Johnathan. Thank you both for making me laugh and being such kind and caring people. I hope you both know the heights you want to reach our possible. I believe in you both.

To Mark. You were there at the beginning and at the end of my time in Oregon and I thought of you as an older brother. A truly sweet guy who has always wanted the best for those around you. I am sorry for letting you down.

To Calie. Thank you for bringing me out of my comfort zone and giving me this opportunity. What a journey it has been and I'm excited for the adventures ahead!

And finally, to my dad. Everything I do, will be for you. The Lad.

FOREWORD

Finding the optimal diet that suits your individual needs isn't meant to be a sprint- it's a marathon. You're allowed to make mistakes, to stumble, to catch your breath, to slow down when you have cramps. Progress is more important than perfection. You can absolutely overcome those bumps in the road. But at the end of the day, you want to finish the marathon and enjoy the journey along the way. You're not an aimless wanderer, you are working towards a goal.

In picking up this book, I understand what that goal is for you. You want to feel alive, with the vibrant health that you deserve, and to find a diet that delivers all of that plus is delicious, simple and affordable. You're looking for a coach who can take your health to the next level. Good news! You've found it in this book you're holding in your hands – *Plant-Based Cooking... Well Kind Of.* I'm glad you're here!

Most people don't realize that I was once an aimless wanderer. They see me as the New York Times bestselling author of *Fiber Fueled* and a gut health expert. That's all great, but you have to know that for the first thirty years of my life, I was a junk food junkie... Hot dogs, cheesesteaks, soda and cold cut subs were my daily routine. I won't lie, I loved them. But they didn't love me back. I gained fifty pounds, had high blood pressure and high anxiety, low self-esteem and low energy. I was thirty, but I felt like I was sixty. I was miserable! And even though I was a doctor, I didn't understand that my diet had caught up to me and my health was suffering as a result.

Then I found the power of a plant-based diet. It allowed me to heal my gut – a great irony considering I spend my days as a gastroenterologist helping people with digestive issues. Up to this point, I hadn't made the connection between my gut and my metabolism, immune system, hormones, cognition and mood. When I healed my gut, these other systems fell into alignment. What followed was effortless fitness. My extra weight melted off, my blood pressure came down, and my anxiety lifted. I felt like myself again, young and energized. In a way, I felt like I had reversed aging. It was incredible.

But you have to understand, I didn't change my diet all at once. It was a process that took years. I made small changes and simple substitutions that would level up my diet. Progress over perfection. Slow and steady.

In many ways, my story was similar to Nic Heffernan, the co-author of this book. We both came from a place of feeling invincible in our youth despite our poor diet. And unfortunately, we both learned the hard way that you can run, but you can't hide. As you'll learn in this book, Nic was a successful athlete who lost his health to a junk food diet. He too came to realize how important nutrition was to his health, but unlike me, he dove right in. Cannonball! Boom. He made the radical change to a plant-based diet all at once... and it's worked for him.

Calie Calabrese, the other co-author of this book, had her own health struggles with leaky gut, autoimmune disease and anxiety. Much like me, she discovered that she had to heal her gut if she wanted to fix her health issues. Once again, the power of plants was crucial to the emergence from her health problems. But it wasn't all at once. She worked through a process. Emphasizing progress over perfection helped her to ultimately reform her health and her life and find happiness.

Calie, Nic and myself each have our own individual stories. So do you. You have your own starting point, your own backstory. You have your own motivations for what you hope to accomplish. And the beauty of *Plant-Based Cooking... Well Kind Of* is that you will have your own journey to better health. This isn't about some rigid plan that shames you for not playing by the rules. This book will meet you where you are and help you chart a path for the future using the power of plants to effortlessly transform your health.

Why plants? They are the definition of anti-inflammatory. Each plant has its own mix of vitamins and minerals helping to nourish your body and give it what it needs. They also have phytochemicals, like quercetin and resveratrol, that are exclusive to plants and have healing properties. There are literally thousands of phytochemicals, many of them contributing to the rainbow of colors that you'll find in the plant world. But my personal favorite is the fiber, which is the preferred food of the microbes living inside of you. If you want a healthy gut, you need to feed your gut microbes with fiber, and there's only one place you'll find fiber... plants.

It really is incredible how powerful this diet can be. It has the potential to protect you from our top killers – heart disease, cancer, stroke, diabetes, chronic kidney disease. As I discuss in my book, *Fiber Fueled*, this is the optimal diet for gut health. It's also the preferred diet in all five Blue Zones, which are the geographic locations across the globe where people have the most longevity. Yes, all of the Blue Zones are at least 90% plant-based, so healthy aging comes with the territory too. And perhaps the best part is that the food is delicious, simple, and affordable. That's what you'll find in this book that you're holding in your hands.

And over time, even the recipes that you don't initially love you'll find that you grow a taste for. Yes, your taste buds come along for the ride!

I've heard many of the concerns with embarking on a plant-based journey. Some worry about protein... Don't worry, the average person will more than meet their protein needs by simply eating a broad diversity of plant foods. Literally all plants contain protein. And if needed, simple modifications can be made by the fitness enthusiast to ensure that their protein needs are met. Both Nic and I lost fat and gained muscle on a plant-based diet.

Others see Instagram photos from paleo and keto enthusiasts and wonder if that's the way to go. It's important to understand that you can look great on the outside, and simultaneously be rotting on the inside. You just may not know it until medical issues show up in the future. Any studies that suggest benefits to these diets are in the short term, ignoring the long-term risks of prioritizing foods that have repeatedly been connected to long term disease risk and shortened life expectancy. Short term gain comes at the expense of long-term pain. Why take that risk? Just know that you will look just as good or better on a plant-based diet, and will simultaneously be consuming the foods offering long term protection and increased life expectancy. Yes, both short term AND long-term gain. Isn't that what we want?

You also don't have to wait for a health scare to be rescued by plants. You can get out ahead of it right now...enjoy a fun, vibrant, energetic life as your healthiest self. The best part? You don't have to focus on restrictive fad diets and deprivation. Instead, you can focus on flavor and fun. When you gravitate to healthy food, you can eat in abundance and without restriction and accomplish all of your health goals.

Whether you are looking to reverse health issues, or you're trying to optimize your health, *Plant-Based Cooking... Well Kind Of* has got your back from start to finish. Human health is a marathon, not a sprint. By following the principles in this book you will both enjoy the journey and turn into your best self in the process.

Onward to health and happiness together!

Will Bulsiewicz, MD MSCI
New York Times bestselling author of *Fiber Fueled*

CONTENTS

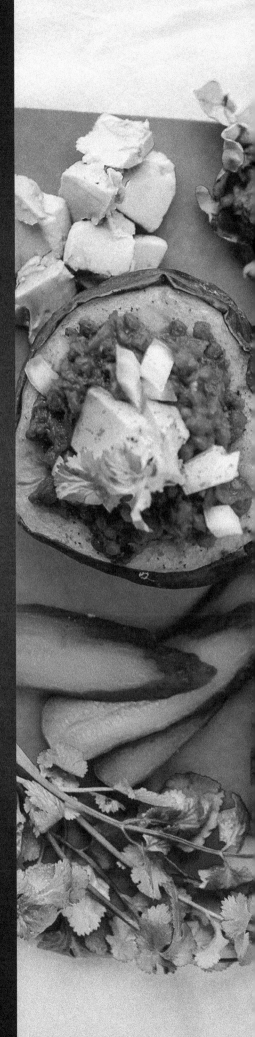

INTRO WHAT'S INSIDE   2

CALIE'S JOURNEY   7

NIC'S JOURNEY   29

OUR JOURNEY   47

BREAKFAST   52

MAIN   68

SIDES   88

GAME DAY & GIRLS NIGHT   106

TREATS   122

SAUCES   130

CALIE VS NIC   138

CALIE'S FAVORITES   146

NIC'S FAVORITES   154

WHAT'S INSIDE, WHY AND HOW TO NAVIGATE THE BOOK

We wrote this book for you guys, not for show. We wanted to help you see that the healing, health and vibrancy we've achieved in our lives is truly available to anyone who simply decides they want it.

We are real, normal people, just like you. We have real struggles, obstacles, and insecurities. We have family and friends who have been unsupportive. We've struggled with money and chosen our health, and plant-based diets with limited cash flow, limited kitchen gadgets, limited cooking knowledge or experience. We've made it work with picky kids. With judgemental mates. We've made it work because we decided we wanted it to work. It's really that simple.

We keep it going because of how it makes us feel. Does it take effort? Yes, especially in the beginning. But like everything...it gets easier the longer you stick with it. And your energy and confidence increase while your need for other people to validate your decisions and journey decrease.

Every photo in this book was taken with our iphones and a small ring light to help light up Nic's apartment. We didn't have make up artists, food stylists, or photo editors. We just used what we had and tried our best to show you what we actually eat in our day to day lives.

We call this book Plant Based...Well Kind Of because it's about progress not perfection. It's about putting more plants on your plate, whether your vegan, vegetarian or a meat lover who is just trying to learn to love vegetables. We include options for transitioning our recipes from vegan or 100% plant-based to adding fish, eggs or other animal protein to make them work for the whole family without having to cook completely separate meals.

Many of the recipes are more of assembly than cooking. Most of them can be made in one pan. The only gadget we ever use besides an oven/stovetop, pots and pans and a can opener is an airfryer, but we also tell you what to do if you don't have one.

You don't have to go out and buy anything special to make these recipes at home. AND we give you lots of ideas for how to change them up if you don't like the veggies we've chosen, if you get bored easily and need variety or if you love to get creative with leftovers. We're all about cooking once and eating two, three or four times off of that time investment.

With that in mind, we've added our favorite pairings to many of the recipes in the book to show you guys what we like to combine to create easy, satisfying, nutrient dense meals with tons of variety. One meal can easily become three just by changing up the pairings that each of us selected. We know you'll have your own favorite combos as well and we can't wait to see what you pair up and how you change things up to make them your own.

While our favorites may not be your favorites, we try to give you an idea of just how stellar a recipe is and where it should rank in your "Ooooh....I can't wait to make this" list with our personal rating system. Let's face it, not liking one or two recipes does not equal hating plant-based food. We all have unique tastes. Some of the recipes Nic loved and Calie...not so much. Some of the recipes Calie loved and Nic took a hard pass. But we guarantee there is something in here for everyone, even the pickiest eaters among you!

And to keep the fun, light-hearted theme strong, we also included our three favorite dishes, plus a Calie vs. Nic cook-off. So you can see some easy ways to change up the same foods and how truly diverse and creative you can get with plant-based meals.

Last, because we know this might be a new way of approaching food and cooking, we included a This for That chart to show you how to swap some of your favorite foods, flavors and cooking techniques so you're plant-based journey can be all about what you get to add in and not about what you feel you have to take out.

We hope you guys have as much fun using this book as we had creating it! We can't wait to see your creations. If you use social media we'd love to see what you're cooking. You can tag us with the hashtags #candnwellness or #calieandnic.

Oh, one more important note. We NEVER cook with white table salt. Every time you see the word salt in our ingredient list, we are referring to Pink Himalayan Sea Salt. We don't get into nutrition science in this book, but google it if you're curious why we choose it and how it's different from processed white table salt.

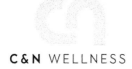

WANT THIS	TRY THIS (GOOD)	OR THIS (BETTER)
Sausage	Plant-based packaged sausage like LightLife or Beyond Meat	Add fennel seeds and sage (main flavors in sausage) to lentils, quinoa, chickpeas or crumbled tofu.
Steak	Have a steak for special occasions like your birthday or Christmas only.	Make a mushroom steak using a portobello mushroom and season like the strips in our "steak" sandwich.
Eggs	Try Just Eggs bottled egg substitute for omelettes and scrambled eggs	Extra Firm Tofu (sprouted and organic) for "fried egg" seasoned with turmeric or silken with turmeric for scrambled or omelettes.
Fish	Tofu seasoned wrapped in or seasoned with seaweed and/or Bragg's seafood seasoning blend	Oyster mushroom stems make great "scallops"
Burgers	Beyond Meat for special occasions, Trader Joe's Hi-Protein veggie burger, Sunshine, Hilary's and Dr. Praegger's Veggie Burgers	Try one of our homemade burger patties
Buffalo Chicken	Wholly Veggie Buffalo Cauliflower Wings	Our Buffalo Cauliflower Wings
Bacon	Smoky Tempeh from LightLife	Make your own tempeh bacon or try eggplant bacon recipes...there are lots online. We haven't perfected our own version, yet. Book 2 :)

4 ■ Plant-Based Cookbook

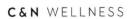
WANT THIS	TRY THIS (GOOD)	OR THIS (BETTER)
Cheese	There are so many great options now. Our favorite brands include: Miyakos, Treeline Violife and Follow Your Heart	Try our homemade nacho cheese recipe or our garlic Parmesan sauce. Nutritional yeast has a "cheesy" flavor and great B vitamins.
Milk	There are lots of super clean 1–2 ingredient dairy free milks now. Oat, Coconut, Hemp, Almond, Macadamia, Cashew, Soy and Rice.	Make your own. It's actually really easy with nothing more than raw nuts, water, a blender and a nut milk bag.
Butter	Earth Balance vegan spreads	Coconut oil Olive oil
Heavy Cream	Melted coconut milk ice cream Non dairy creamers like Califia, Silk, Laird, Ripple, and PicNik	Canned coconut milk
Mayonaisse	Veganise or Just Mayo	Make your own. There are lots of easy recipes online.
Honey	Agave Nectar, Brown Rice Syrup and Real 100% Maple Syrup	
Ice Cream	Some of our favorite brands that offer plant-based ice creams include: So Delicious, Halo Top, Enlightened, Ben & Jerry's, Talenti, Rice Dream, Oatly	Make your own with frozen fruit and coconut milk or cashew milk

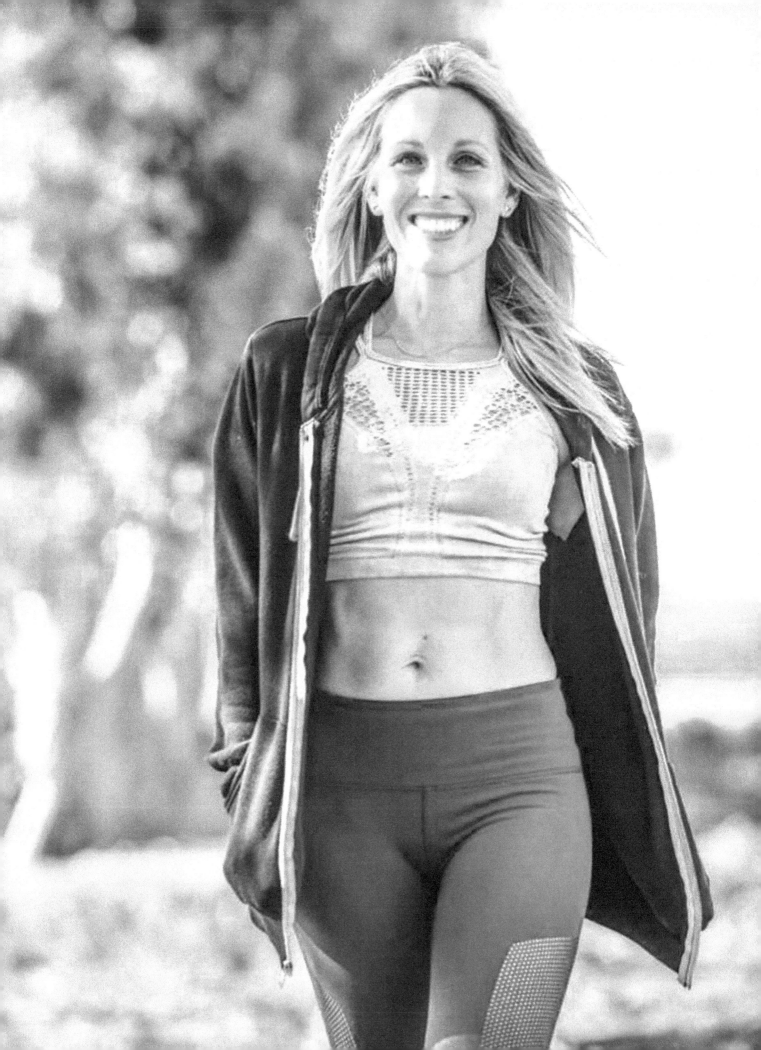

CALIE'S JOURNEY

Where do I even begin? I think by reminding myself that hindsight is truly 20/20. It's only with the mindset I've developed over the last four years that I can look back on the experiences that have shaped my life and see them with absolute gratitude. While there was definitely a time where I would have described my life as hard, unfair, even miserable...I genuinely mean it 100% when I say I would go back and live it all again to get to be the person I am today and experiencing the life I'm experiencing.

I now understand that these things happened to me. They don't define me. And they didn't happen to me...but happened for me. They were preparing me, teaching me, molding me into the person I needed to become to live out my purpose. But again...it took hindsight and a lot of work to get to a place where I can see things that way. So let's look back...why? Because often (almost always) when I share my lifestyle choices with people now, I hear "But you don't understand? You've never... (insert excuse...negative mindset...victim mentality)" OR "I would do that if...(insert circumstance we claim is outside of our control that is really simply outside of our comfort zone.)" I know because I was that girl... for 39 of my current 43 years.

Childhood

I grew up in a very close-knit Italian family, the oldest of 3 (who would later become 5 with different dads). I had 10 cousins, who were more like brothers and sisters. My parents got divorced when I was 6 and my mom moved to New York with her new husband when I was 9, leaving me, my brother and my sister with my dad back in Cleveland, Ohio.

My dad owned an Italian pizza place called Bobby Cal's. We lived in an apartment above it in a small Italian

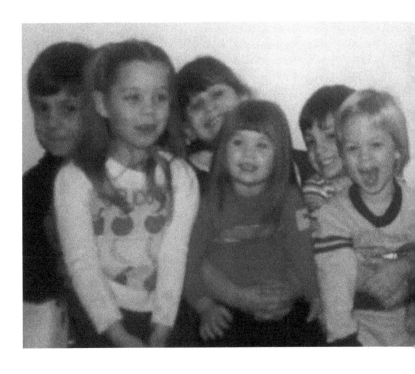

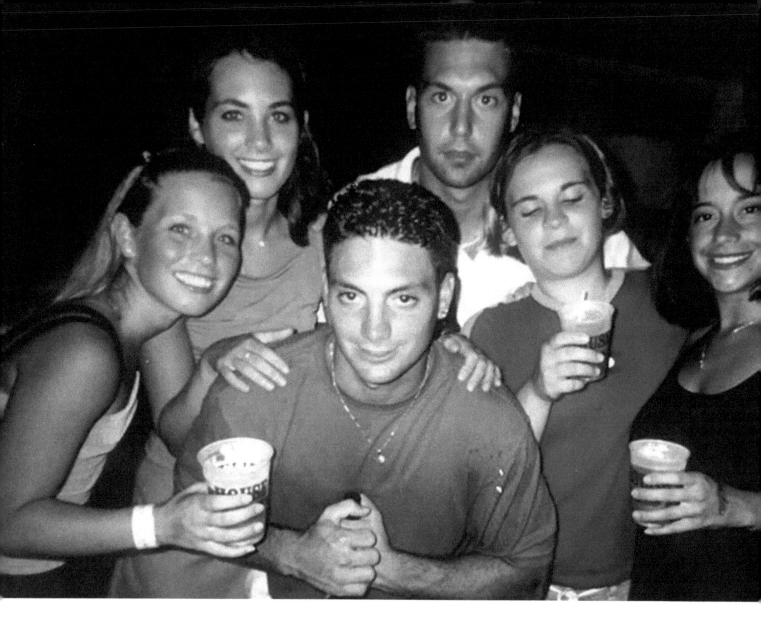

neighborhood known as Collinwood...we just called it "The Neighborhood." Everyone knew everyone. And everyone definitely knew my dad's restaurant. I went to a Catholic Elementary school down the street from our restaurant and most of what I remember relates to family, helping my dad with the restaurant and with my brother and sister and food.

Sometimes we were financially stable and sometimes we struggled. My dad was stressed, anxious and honestly...angry a lot. He loved us, that was never a question. And we were always surrounded by family helping out. My grandparents helped raise us and my aunts were always there for us too.

We grew up fast. We knew everything that was going on whether they intended for us to or not. I mean, we're Italian. We love to talk! And kids are amazingly perceptive. We all worked in the restaurant. Making salads, chopping veggies and cutting up salami (in triangles so it could be laid in pretty circles on the antipasto salad), mixing vats of dressing in giant jugs that were taller than us, stirring sauce and rolling dough balls to rise for the day's pizzas. We answered phones, took orders, rang the register and went on deliveries with my dad to some of the big offices and factories in "the neighborhood." That's just how it was. Everyone pitched in. And when Dad went out, or next door to the Green Lantern for drinks and time with his friends, I babysat, for Autumn and Bobby... although let's be honest...by babysat, I mean called the bar and told on them or got into trouble with them.

I don't remember eating breakfast as a kid. Maybe toast with butter and jelly sometimes. I do remember sitting in the little green and silver metal chairs outside the principal's office at school waiting for one of my dad's employees, usually Sal, to deliver our lunch. Food from the restaurant. On our birthdays, it was always pizza with our age scripted in pepperoni. (We were pretty popular in the school lunchroom on our birthdays!) Sometimes my dad made dinner, sometimes he asked me to make it, most of the time we just ate from the restaurant. When we moved away from "the neighborhood" because my dad felt it wasn't safe for us anymore...we ate a lot of peanut butter sandwiches and pickles waiting for my dad to get home from work with dinner.

I'm sure we ate vegetables at some point, but all I can remember consistently eating from the veggie family was our Sunday dinner salad at grandma's house. The whole family got together at my grandma's house pretty much every Sunday of my life until I went away to college. It was always pasta, homemade tomato sauce (which I guess counted as a vegetable despite being prepared with a pound of Crisco!!!!), white Italian bread and butter, our dinner salad of romaine, tomatoes, cucumbers and homemade Italian dressing and RC Cola...my grandpa's favorite pop (soda for those of you who aren't from Ohio.)

My dad had a temper, and anxiety, and I remember feeling anxious, scared and stressed out a lot. I probably couldn't use those words to describe my feelings at the time, but I was highly sensitive and I learned to be a people pleaser at a very young age because it was the best way to keep the peace and feel safe.

I loved to read. It was my escape. And I decided at a very young age that I wouldn't live in Cleveland forever (maybe because I got to experience other places through books and my mom moving every few years with her husband's job). I knew that school and education were my way out. We didn't have a lot of money. Everyone I'd ever known was born and died in Cleveland and no one I knew dreamed of leaving. But I was leaving, and school was how I would do it.

School was where I felt safe and happy. I was good at it. No one yelled. And I knew exactly how to control my day. Do my work. Follow directions and things would go smoothly. Easy. Much easier than controlling the environment at

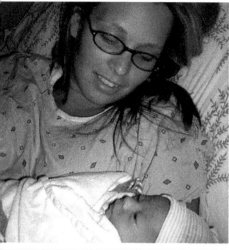
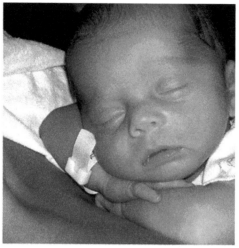
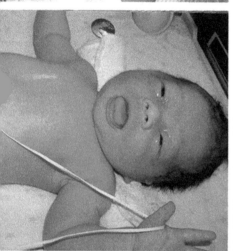
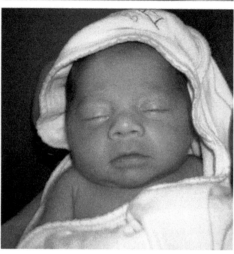

home. And when I needed to escape...I had my books and my drawing. I worked hard from middle school.... straight through high school and I was eventually accepted into my dream school. Miami University (not University of Miami in sunny Florida...I wasn't a big dreamer back then guys... getting out of Cleveland and going to college was already huge!) Miami University, in Oxford, Ohio. Five hours from home. Far enough that I couldn't get surprise visits and close enough that it wasn't too scary.

I applied for scholarships, got financial aid and it was a state school so it was doable for me (with students loans I'm literally still paying off today) since my dad had filed bankruptcy that year and couldn't afford to pay for college.

I don't ever remember thinking about my health outside of my weight during all that time. I do remember thinking about my size. I remember trying to eat to be skinny. Trying to make weight for the crew team in high school. Feeling really insecure about my Italian butt and thighs (it was the age of Kate Moss...not Jennifer Lopez and the Kardashians') and my brother saying "boom ba boom ba" when I walked past him in reference to the size of my booty. Not great for a girl's self-esteem even though he thought it was hilarious.

I remember dieting, starving myself on Sunday's and holiday's so I could eat as much pasta and bread as I wanted at my one meal and living off a steady diet of chocolate chip cookies (we called them 'better than sex cookies' at our Catholic all girls high school even though none of us actually knew that from experience!) and French fries with ranch dressing for lunch, bagels and pasta before regattas and weekends driving through Burger King ordering the chicken sandwich with extra-cheese, large fries and a fountain coke. Fountain coke was my favorite. Fountain coke and cheese! My go-to after school snack was graham crackers dipped in vanilla ice cream and that all seemed normal to me. It's how all of my friends ate too. When you're 16 and working out twice a day with your Crew team, you can do that, and it doesn't show up on your body. But inside my body and my brain...I had no idea the damage I was doing and the consequences I would suffer in the coming years because of it.

College

College! Freedom! Total opportunity to create my dream life. I applied as an architecture major, but when I got to orientation, I found out that all art majors had to live on the "alternative" campus. Picture me...5" 100 lbs. blonde bob cut to just above my shoulders, barely wore any makeup (didn't really know how to do make up or hair since I grew up with my dad), khaki shorts, white t-shirt, plaid long sleeve, shirt over it, white keds and simple gold studs in my ears. I walk into orientation and literally every person in the room is dressed in head to toe black, Doc Martin's are the shoe of choice, they have tattoos, black hair, pink hair, green hair, thick black eyeliner (guys and girls), face piercings. Nice. Friendly. But I stood out like a sore thumb.

> **That was one of the first major life decisions I remember making based on fear and it was a pattern I would repeat over and over for the next 20 years.**

The quiet, shy girl, who keeps the peace and keeps her head down suddenly had all eyes on her. I cried and within 2 hours told my advisor I was dropping architecture as my major. I was terrified to dorm on that campus. To this day I find myself telling people I switched majors because architecture was too much math and science, which is half true. The course curriculum shocked me on orientation day. But I would have toughed it out. The truth is...I didn't want to live with the art majors because it was way out of my comfort zone. I wanted to be on the regular campus.

That was one of the first major life decisions I remember making based on fear and it was a pattern I would repeat over and over for the next 20 years.

I eventually settled on journalism as my major after an English teacher complimented my story writing skills and suggested I give a few journalism and writing classes a try. (Universe nudge #1...not sure this book would be in your hands right now if it wasn't for that teacher and her encouragement...I wish I could remember her name.)

For a long time, I thought my 4.5 years at Miami were the best years of my life. I loved my friends, I loved my classes, I worked hard to put myself through school and I was finally able to date. Oh yeah, my dad didn't let me date at all in high school. But I was also never myself. I was still the girl trying to fit in, fly under the radar, keep the peace and I was still a massive people pleaser. My roommates called the shots...or my boyfriend and I carefully crafted my personality to fit in and be accepted despite being in a very different place than most of my friends.

I didn't realize what I was doing at the time, but it was taking a huge toll on my self-esteem. Miami was an expensive school you guys and almost everyone was Greek (in a fraternity or sorority), which I couldn't afford to be a part of (and honestly hated the 1 year I participated). I was the poor kid. I didn't have my parents credit card. All of the money I made went to pay my tuition and living expenses. I didn't really have money for food so when I moved out of the dorms my junior year I literally lived off a giant box (like a moving wardrobe box) of canned and boxed soups, tuna and mac-n-cheese my mom sent me. The little extra money I had I spent on Natty Light and the occasional McDonald's hangover meal or late night Bagel & Deli (steamed bagel sandwich with about a pound of meat and cheese on them), oh and my morning 30 oz Mountain Dew on the way to my 8 a.m. classes.

> **My roommates called the shots... or my boyfriend and I carefully crafted my personality to fit in and be accepted despite being in a very different place than most of my friends.**

I gained the Freshman 15 then lost it. Then gained it. Then lost it. My weight fluctuated heavily throughout college (ranging from a size 2 to an 8 at 5'2") and I had my first full blown panic attack my senior year. Oh, and I was constantly sick. I had chronic sinus infections. Chronic bladder infections. I was put on Allegra-D my sophomore year to try to control the sinus issues, which I stayed on until I was 30 and I took a minimum of 3 antibiotic prescriptions a year if not more. I also started taking birth control at the advice of the school doctor.

By the time I graduated and headed off to Chicago to work in a PR agency on Michigan avenue I had learned how to control my weight by controlling my portions and exercising, but my diet was still seriously lacking in nutrients and my anxiety and breathing issues were rapidly getting worse.

My Twenties

Before you think I was just miserable all of the time, let me say that I wasn't. I was struggling with anxiety. I was definitely a people pleaser and worried A LOT about what other people thought of me. But in some ways, that really served me. I was determined to remain independent. To never have to go home to Cleveland or move in with my parents. I had a shit ton of debt, but I was motivated as fuck to pay it off.

I got a job just before graduation by showing up at a sales recruiting seminar I saw on a job board at school for business majors. I was an English/Journalism major, but they were hiring for the local newspaper. So I printed out my resume, a bunch of writing samples from class and my internship at the Hamilton Daily News (where I wrote about things like the biggest tomato at the town festival) and I showed up in a suit and asked the sales recruiter to connect me with someone who hired writers. I never thought it would actually work, but at least I'd be able to say I tried. And next thing I knew...I had a job! And six months later...I quit that job. I packed up my turquoise blue Ford Ranger and I moved to Chicago. Nowhere to live. No job. But I was 22. I'd figure it out!

I was determined to remain independent. To never have to go home to Cleveland or move in with my parents. I had a shit ton of debt, but I was motivated as fuck to pay it off.

My boyfriend lived there, most of my college friends and roommates had moved there and that's where I wanted to be. My journalism job at the Cincinnati Enquirer barely paid my bills and PR jobs used a lot of the same skills but paid significantly more. The only problem...I had no experience. No internships. Just a desire to make more money and live close to my boyfriend and my friends. I was rejected at interview after interview. Time and money were running out and I was seriously thinking I was going to have to move home to Cleveland.

And then one weekend everything changed. I was staying on my friend Lisa's couch and she was throwing a party. I remember drinking a beer on her back patio and meeting this guy named Neal. (Universe moment #2) Guess where Neal worked guys? At one of the largest PR agencies in Chicago. Ketchum Public Relations. We started talking and by the end of the night he had a copy of my resume and promised to give it to his boss and see if he could get me an interview. (For all of you wondering...nothing ever happened between Neal and I....other than we ended up working at the same PR agency!)

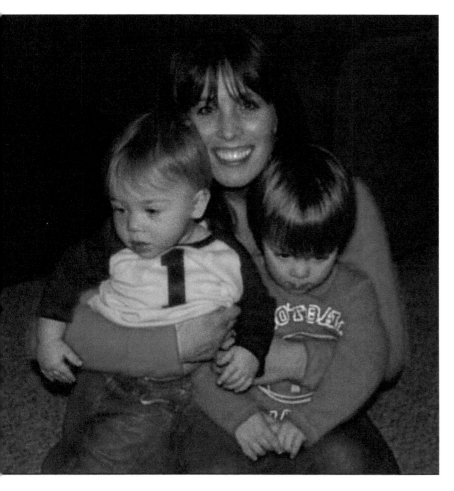

I got the interview and I prepared for that interview for days. I took everything I had learned from my rejections and I went in more confident than I'd ever felt. At the end of the interview Michelle told me they didn't have any openings at the moment. They had already hired all of their interns for the year, but she took my resume and writing test to her boss and they created an internship for me. Yup, I was starting as an intern being paid hourly, but after 3 months, if I did well, I could be moved to salary.

That same week, after wearing out my welcome on couches across the city, I was sitting at breakfast at a small deli in the suburb where my boyfriend and his parents lived. I was mildly hungover from a night out when I felt a tap on my leg. The cutest little blonde 2-year-old girl (Universe moment #3) was standing next to me and she struck up a conversation with me. We talked for a few minutes and I had her laughing...I can't remember about what...when her mom walked over and commented on how unusual her daughter's behavior was with me. She apparently was normally very shy. (She must have sensed her kind.) The woman jokingly asked if I babysat and being desperate for a job and money I said yes, I do. She looked at me surprised and said really...my nanny just quit, and I could really use some help with me kids (she had 3).

We ended up working out a deal where she allowed me to live in the guest bedroom of their house, in exchange for my help getting the kids ready for school in the morning before I took the train to work in the city, and my help with the kids after work and on the weekends. I now had a job and a beautiful place to live while I saved up some money again and got back on my feet. I don't think I truly appreciated how amazing that opportunity was back then, and I honestly can't even remember the family's name. I felt so unworthy and embarrassed at my circumstances that I spent most of the time hiding in my room and just doing what she asked of me instead of truly embracing the experience. I also got to a point where I felt resentful that I had to rush home after work and spent so much time on the train back and forth to the city. I was ready to live independent and free, but at some level I felt like an indentured servant. I had a bad attitude. Instead of appreciating the gift I'd been given, instead of saving money, getting to know the family, staying in touch with them, I saved up as much money as I could as fast as I could, I got the offer for the full-time job at the end of the 3 months and I got the hell out. Real nice, Calie. I think I did send her a thank you letter about a year later, but I never even visited the kids again. I was super selfish and in a mindset of I've endured so much...I'm ready to live my life for me.

There are lots of times in my life where little guardian angels were placed in my path, but I didn't see them for what they were at the time. I look back at them now and I have insane gratitude. I've spent hours writing thank you letters that were never sent (but needed to be written nonetheless), sending light and love to those people and reflecting on how life changing so many of them were. It's not the same as telling them to their face or in the moment, but it was a really powerful and positive experience for me on my healing journey. But I'm getting ahead of myself...

Let's get back to Michigan Avenue and Ketchum Public Relations....

Independence and Marriage

I fucking loved my PR job. I lived in a beautiful condo in Lincoln Park, rode the L to work. Jumped out of bed at 5 a.m. every day to get ready and get in by 7 a.m. so we could send out client's daily news updates and how we were using the stories to pitch their businesses, products and services to the media. It was called the News Engine and the team that worked on it was really close.

In addition to working together, we generally ate meals together, met up in the breakroom for midday foosball matches with a diet coke and Snackwell's fat free cookies, played on a beach volleyball league together, a 16" softball league together and enjoyed Miller Friday's in the office (beer & snacks on the house from our client...Miller...starting at 4 p.m.)

We worked hard and played harder. I remember very clearly walking down Michigan Avenue looking at the beach and the lake and thinking...I did it...I live here! I love it! I'm sooooo happy!

And that's where I met my ex-husband. He was the account manager for our team. We were both dating other people when we first met, and we started out as friends for about 2 years. Then one day, we were both single at the same time. I won't go into all the details of dating and marriage, but here's what's important to know.

We got engaged after just two months. A sure sign that we were both very unhealthy individuals at the time. He wanted to put a ring on it before I figured out who he really was and at 25, I was one of the last of my friends to get engaged. I had just broken up with my boyfriend of 4 years and I actually thought...I'm going to be so old by the time I get married. I have to meet someone, date for a few years, get engaged. I'll be mid-30s before I have kids! And then, there he was...proposing to me over cold Wendy's in his Oak Park apartment in our pajamas while I was sick because "the ring was burning a hole in his pocket". And there I was saying yes...focused on the excitement of a wedding and not being alone and not having to wait until my 30s to have kids.

Our engagement lasted a year and a half and during that time I was given ample reason and opportunity to call it off. I wanted to call it off. I thought about it all of the time. So why didn't I?

1. I was afraid of hurting him.
2. How embarrassing would that be? What would people think? We'd already sent out wedding invitations!
3. His family would hate me.
4. We'd waste a lot of money we'd spent on the wedding already and we were paying for it ourselves.
5. We lived together. Where would I go?

I tried to talk to a few friends about it and everyone said the same thing. "You just have cold feet." But I knew in my gut it was more than that. I knew something was terribly off. I had such a bad feeling.

The day of the wedding I vividly remember feeling sick all morning. Not bride excited, but terrified. My two best friends from high school showed up at the hotel to help me get ready. I was standing there in my gorgeous gown that I loved, trying to be excited and hopeful that it was all going to be ok. And suddenly I was screaming...."get it off....get the dress off...I'm gonna be sick!" And two minutes later I was bent over the toilet in my corset throwing up my insides. That should have been the final straw. I still had time to back out. But we blamed it on nerves, excitement, the heat and the corset! And so I got married that day against the prompting of my gut. And I stayed unhappily married for 14 years.

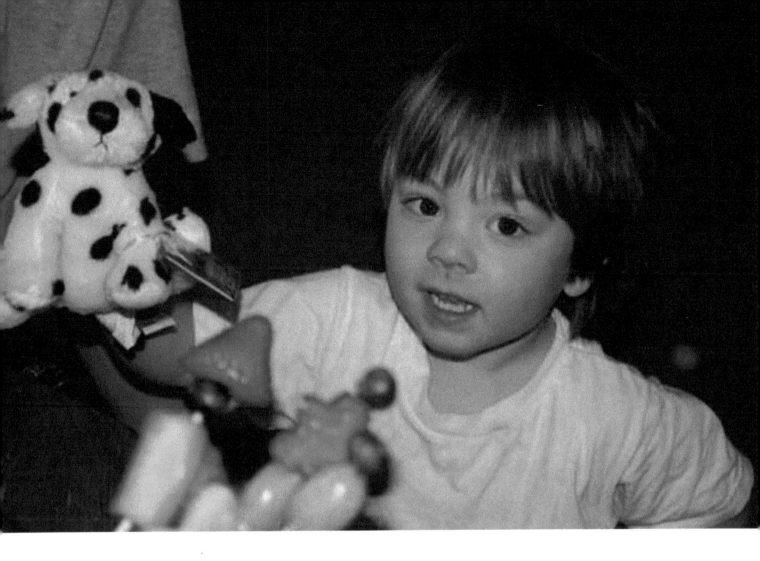

We had some fun moments. But if you look back on the whole of our marriage... we fought a lot. We didn't really engage with each other. Red flags popped up all of the time that something was wrong. He was always angry. Never physically abusive toward me. In fact, most of the time his anger was directed at himself. But he would rage. And just like in my childhood, I learned to become who I thought he needed me to be to try and keep the peace. But it never worked.

I desperately tried to figure out how to make him happy. But you guys, happiness comes from within. You can't create it for someone else and no one can create it for you. I wish 25-year-old Calie had known that. But then again...she was on a journey and it was worth it!

On our 1-year wedding anniversary we stood next to a lighthouse in Maine after arguing for 3 hours because we got lost and he was furious with himself for being so dumb. It had been an absolutely miserable day and he was in the apologizing phase that always came after one of his tantrums and for the first time ever I said "something has to change or we aren't going to make it to year 2." Nothing changed and we "made it" for 13 more years.

Over the course of the next 4 years, we were pregnant 3 times. First, we had our oldest son, Kade. He was born at 36 weeks and 3 days and spent 5 days in the hospital trying to gain weight and overcome jaundice. His delivery was traumatic for both of us.

The quick version is while I was in the hospital being checked for early labor, I had a massive minute long contraction that sent Kade's little body into distress. I remember laying in the bed in some pain and discomfort when alarms started going off and nurses came running into the room. They were talking to each other and checking machines and trying to stick IVs into the top of my hand. We kept asking what was going on and they kept telling us there was not time to explain. They got the IV in my vein, injected something into it and watched the machines. When they saw the response, they were looking for they explained that Kade's heart rate had dropped to a dangerously low level. They

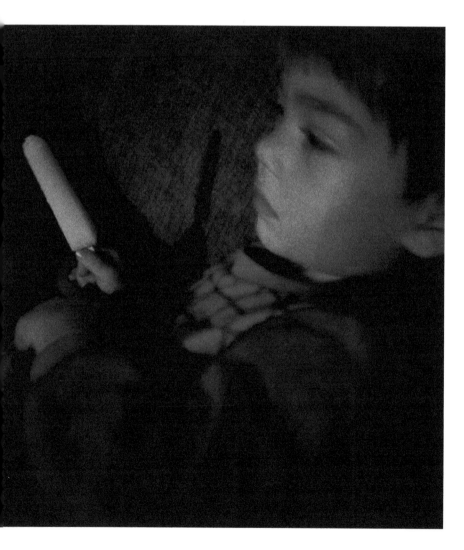

injected me with something to help bring it up and he responded. I was definitely in labor, but they decided to give me more drugs to stop it so his body and mine could rest until my doctor could come in in the morning. His heart rate dropped again later that night and they repeated the same exercise.

That's when my doctor was called in and I was given another drug to start my labor back up. It was time to get Kade out. The only problem. My body did not like the double dose of meds that helped Kade's heart rate. Now we couldn't get mine down. They put me on oxygen and rolled in a crash cart. A doctor was hanging out to the side with it. I looked at it, the nurse looked at me and said, "just in case."

Fear gripped my entire body. I couldn't breathe. I looked at my then husband and said "pray". I genuinely thought I was going to die.

Obviously, I didn't. Kade was face up instead of down and he was stuck. No matter what position I pushed from, we couldn't get him out. They finally gave us two choices. Try the vacuum to get a good grip, flip him, and hope I could push him out OR emergency C-section. We opted for the vacuum and Kade come out on the next push. Bruised, cone shaped head. But otherwise doing great.

When they told me he had to stay in the hospital because of his jaundice levels, but I was being released I lost my shit. I refused to leave. Told them I was going to sit in the hallway all day and all night. Have I mentioned I'm stubborn? Thankfully, things were slow at the hospital that week. They couldn't feed me or provide any care for me, but they gave me a room so I could stay and nurse him the last 3 days until he was released to come home with me.

Looking back, I'm confident that some of the drugs were part of what exploded the inflammation bomb in my body and caused the insane symptoms I was about to experience for the next 4 years and the same for Kade who struggled with chronic breathing issues from infancy, a seriously weak immune system and horrible eczema.

At this point, my biggest health scares, other than Kade's delivery, were one high cholesterol reading despite being thin, one abnormal pap smear and a few anxiety attacks.

My recovery from Kade's birth was not smooth. I ended up in the hospital for a potential blood clot in my lungs, which turned out to be a panic attack and misread Xray. But resulted in 48 hours of monitoring and lots of tests and dye injections into my veins. I didn't sleep. At all. My anxiety was unbearable. I set alarms to check that Kade was breathing. I was terrified to be alone. I was afraid to fall asleep because I wasn't sure I'd wake up and my marriage was the worst it had ever been. I had zero interest in my husband. I was totally consumed with keeping Kade and myself alive. I had no libido and we were already struggling pre-baby so there was that. His ego took a major hit. He felt ignored and neglected and even jealous.

Four months postpartum I found out I was pregnant again! And I lost my shit! I was absolutely terrified. I had decided we were done having kids and now I was pregnant before I was even healed.

Eight weeks later, getting used to the idea of another baby, I headed to my OBGYN with my 6 month old (but not my husband...he said he had to work...to be fair, I said I was fine to go alone even though I wasn't) to hear the new baby's heartbeat for the first time. It was our 12-week appointment. They sent me to the bathroom to pee in a cup before I went in for the ultrasound and when I sat down to do that....I started gushing blood. Gushing! Sorry I know it's graphic.

Over the course of the next two weeks, I went back and forth every 3 days for blood work. My hormone levels continued coming down, I continued bleeding and I painfully lost the baby in a natural miscarriage at home in isolation. I was so embarrassed that I had cried over being pregnant. I felt totally ashamed and I wouldn't talk to anyone about it. My husband continued working. I continued taking care of Kade and that was that.

When my maternity leave was up, I couldn't trust Kade's care to a stranger or a daycare center. My anxiety was too high. I had to be in control at all times. But my husband wouldn't let me quit working. So I found a freelance job, working in PR from home for my old boss from Ketchum in Chicago. She had started her own agency.

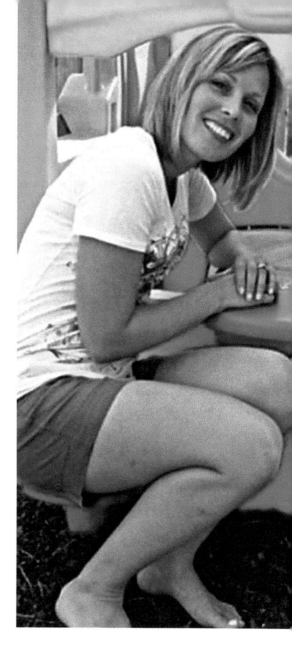

We found a new normal that included both of us focusing on the baby and our jobs and watching TV and drinking wine every night until bedtime. We tried to make things work or make them better. We had good weeks and bad weeks. Good days and bad days. And then we decided to have another baby.

During this time, I was diagnosed with low thyroid and put on the lowest dose of levothyroxine. This was after a lot of doctor's visits. And I'll share something very personal with you guys. I desperately wanted my marriage to work. I wanted to make him happy and I wanted to be happy. I went to counseling. We went to counseling. I went to doctors and tried to figure out why I had no libido and why I had so much anxiety. And at one of those appointments I distinctly remember the doctor looking me in the eye and saying, there's nothing physically wrong with you. Is your marriage happy? And I looked her in the eye, lied and said yes, very.

Despite our issues, we got pregnant with our second son, Jake. That delivery turned out very similar to the first one. I went into labor at exactly 36 weeks and

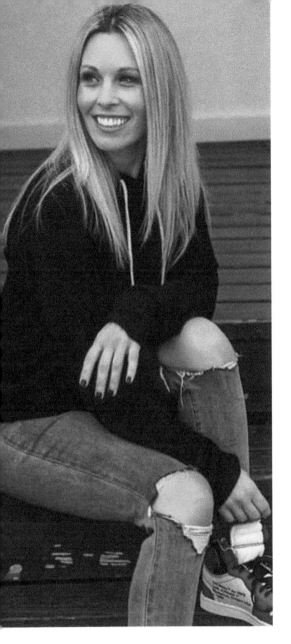

3 days. But this time, the main complication was that my test epidural run went up and numbed my heart and lungs instead of down to numb my abdomen. The nurse told me I would have died if she hadn't stayed in the room and been there to give me medicine to reverse the effect.

So Jake was born early, naturally, at 7 lbs. 11 oz and the doctor said one more day and I never would have got his big body out of my tiny body. But he was healthy. Well for the most part. But like his big brother, he was constantly sick from day 1. At 6 weeks he had so much mucus, it blocked his airways and my mom had to call an ambulance while I was at my OBGYN checkup because he turned blue.

He had chronic sinus infections his first year, unheard of for babies and in an effort to nurse him and care for two constantly sick little guys, I became the sickest I had ever been. I lost a ton of weight. I never slept. I started reacting to foods unpredictably and breaking out in rashes all over my body. My anxiety was no longer inconvenient. It was disruptive to my life and all encompassing. I couldn't work. I couldn't eat if I was alone. I cried all the time. We were in the pediatrician's office at least once a week and I was in and out of doctor's offices just as much. Was my marriage still shit. I think so, but honestly, it was all a blur. We weren't living. We were surviving.

This final straw! Or so I thought…

When Jake was about 16 weeks old, I decided to let go a little, leave the boys with their dad and head to a girl's night out.

It was a great night for the first few hours. I wasn't consciously thinking about all the things I needed to do, I was gonna pump and dumb after the party because Jake had enough milk for the night, so I was thoroughly enjoying the taco bar and margaritas and the adult conversation and then I noticed my stomach was itching.

I scratched it a few times and then my forearm started to itch. I looked down at it and there was a small red welt. I excused myself to go to the bathroom and lifted my shirt. A few red welts were on my stomach too.

Suddenly I felt hot all over. Like an instant fever came over me and I couldn't breathe. Now my heart is racing, and I'm surrounded by people. Some are close friends and some I don't really know at all. I grab my phone from my purse and head to the bathroom to call my doctor. What did I eat? Were there nuts? (I'm not allergic to nuts but in my state of anxiety I always had a fear that I was going to develop a nut allergy...anxiety isn't rational guys!)

I explained the symptoms to my doctor once he called me back from the emergency line. His advice. Take some Benadryl and see if it calms down and if not...go to the ER.

> My face is bright red and tears are streaming down my face.

I find Jen in the kitchen and ask her if she has any Benadryl. Obviously, she asks what's going on and I explain that I think I might be having an allergic reaction to something I ate. But she's a counselor and she can tell I'm in panic mode. She finds our friend Jamie, who is a nurse, and some children's Benadryl, but by now, everyone knows something is going on. Conversation has stopped and all eyes are on the three of us. I'm so mortifyingly embarrassed. My face is bright red and tears are streaming down my face.

I take the Benadryl, we sit at the table and everyone is talking to me, asking about what happened and being super sweet and supportive, but I'm still embarrassed. I feel like I hijacked everyone's girl's night with my drama and ruined the evening for them all. The Benadryl makes me sleepy and after about 45 minutes my heart rate calms, the welts are gone, and I start to breathe a little easier.

The next morning, I was taking care of the boys and praying for an answer. I felt like I just couldn't go on living like this. I got the mail and sat down with my coffee to flip through a clipper magazine (you know, those coupon junk mail books) because I just needed a distraction and the boys were happily watching Doodle Bops.

The first page I opened to was an ad for a new chiropractor in town. Down the left side of the page was a giant list of symptoms she treated and the first word on the list was ANXIETY. I knew in my gut immediately that I was supposed to call her. (Universe nudge #4)

I made an appointment for that week with Dr. Jana Joshu and it changed my life!

I arrived with my boys filled with hope, fear, anxiety and a lot of questions. She sat me down in her office and she never even adjusted me...she just asked me questions and listened to my story. The story of both boys' births, of my struggles, of my sudden food sensitivities, of my stress, of my marriage. And then she said the sentence I'll never forget. It's the sentence that gave me back my life, my health and set me on a path to finding my purpose in this world.

She said...I'm going to teach you how to eat and it's going to change your life!

I looked at the Ritz Crackers my boys were gnawing on, suddenly embarrassed...I looked at her, and I said, "I'm ready!"

Getting My Life and Health Back and Paying It Forward

Dr. Jana delivered on her promise. Within a few weeks of starting her nutrition program my panic attacks had completely stopped. I still had some feelings of anxiousness, but I had control over it. No more ER visits and I started sleeping at night.

Within 3 months of changing how we ate; I was off my allergy medicine and both boys were taken off their allergy medicine by the allergist. Jake was also able to come off his reflux medicine. Did I mention he had uncontrollable reflux and threw up all the time? Well, yeah, he had that.

I was so fascinated by the power of food to completely change my mood, my brain and all of our health. I couldn't believe how fast it helped. I started a blog called Broccoli Cupcake to chronicle and share my journey and everything I was learning. It kept me accountable, writing the posts helped me retain everything I was learning, and it gave me a way to connect with other women who were on similar journeys or experiencing similar struggles.

From there, I enrolled at the Institute for Integrative Nutrition to get my Holistic Health Coaching Certification and I eventually opened a barre studio in my town with my best friend, Jen.

Studio 3 Fitness became a place for me to share my passion for all things health. Yes, we taught barre and other workouts, but we also hosted nutrition workshops, shared recipe ideas, and taught essential oils classes. We built a community and for the first time in a long time I started to feel joy again.

Studio 3 was my happy place...but I still had health and marriage struggles.

I can't get lupus. I'm a fucking health coach!

Another sleepless night...tossing and turning...trying to find a position where my back and hips don't hurt. The boys will be up soon. Have I even slept? Just get up and make coffee Calie. It will work itself out like it always does. I roll to the side of the bed to push myself up and the pain shoots up my back! Fuck...I can't unbend my legs! I flip on my back and try to pull myself up with my abs. The pain escalates and my body doesn't budge. Stay calm Calie...you're just stiff. Stretch. I try to pull my knee into my chest, but the pain is too intense. I can barely move my leg. And I have to pee. I shake my husband who is sleeping soundly. Hey...I need your help. I can't get up. "What?" I can't get up. I need you to help me out of the bed...I have to pee, and I can't move my legs. I'm not even 35 and I can't get out of bed on my own. I make a doctor's appointment and they send me to a rheumatologist. I have all the precursors to lupus. My inflammation levels are through the roof. But I eat healthy. I'm a size 2. I teach fitness classes and I've stopped eating processed foods and sugar. My diet is real food, paleo, like everyone suggested. I'm the healthiest I've ever been. My allergies are gone, and my anxiety has been so much better. How can this be happening? The doctor assures me that I don't actually have lupus...yet. We don't need to start medication, but we need to monitor the situation. We will do blood work every 3 months so we can decide when it's time to start medicine. The decision seemed final. It wasn't would I need lupus medication...it was when.

I don't accept it! I know the power of food. I start to research anti-inflammatory diets and I keep coming across the healing power of plants. I decided to double down on my veggie intake, cut my meat consumption significantly. I talked to my ex about going vegan or vegetarian, but he was an extremely picky eater and he was not supportive of that idea. But I found ways to make it work. I used meat to flavor food, but not as the main dish. I cooked meat for him and the boys and opted for extra servings of veggies for myself. I also cut my nightly wine intake significantly. Within about 6 months my inflammation levels came down and my joint pain subsided. After 9 months, my doctor released me from regular blood testing and told me I didn't need to come back unless the pain came back. I was thrilled. Once again...food had been the answer.

I continued running my studio for the next couple years, eating what I would call a plant-based diet. Super heavy on the veggies, lots of berries, dark chocolate as my main treat and meat occasionally. I was still eating eggs pretty regularly but hardly ever had red meat and I definitely looked and felt the best I had since my boys were born.

Life was calm for a while after that. We sold our house, bought land to build our dream house on a cul-de-sac one house down from our boys best friends on a street loaded with kids their age. We moved into a condo while the construction was being finished and for the first time in almost 14 years, I felt happy and hopeful. My ex and I were getting along the best we ever had. He was working from home running a marketing agency of his own. I was running my studio. We were homeschooling the boys and enjoying tons of time with our travel baseball family. I dared to believe that we just might be happy.

Heath's arrest

Until October 9...

That was the day my ex-husband was arrested in a prostitution sting. It was also the day I found out my husband of 14 years was a sex addict.

The next 6 months were a total blur. I was in shock.

Too shocked, too scared, too paralyzed, too confused to think or make a decision. He took the lead on what happened next. We started going to counseling, together and individually. I still didn't know everything. The counselor wanted to wait until he felt I was ready to hear the full truth and he needed more time to help Heath get to a place where he could remember and tell me everything.

I remember worrying about him. Him and the boys. He kept making comments that made me wonder if he'd hurt himself. The shame seemed to be torturing him. All I could think about was worse case scenarios because my safety and security had been completely rocked. I imagined finding him. I imagined the boys finding him. I imagined having to tell the boys their dad was gone. I was paralyzed with fear and I had no idea what to do. I knew our marriage had problems, I honestly had always wanted to leave, but this was beyond anything I ever could have imagined.

Late November rolled around, and the counselor decided it was time for what they called the Discovery session. I was told to find a friend to drive me to and from the appointment. They would not allow me to drive myself home after. I was told to prepare for 3 hours, but nothing could prepare me for what I was about to learn.

It was absolutely gut wrenching. I cried. I screamed. I sat on the floor holding my knees to my chest trying to breathe. Trying to understand how all of that could be going on for 14 years and how I had no idea. How was there not one good year. Not one good memory. Everything was tainted. I felt like I would never recover.

After that, things got worse for me physically and emotionally. I tried to put on a happy face and go through the healing counseling work. I thought I needed to keep the family together for the boys. And honestly, for Heath. I was still afraid he would hurt himself. I pretended to be ok.

But I felt like I was dying inside. I secretly went to multiple doctor's appointments. Something was wrong. I had read a bunch of books from the counselor that talked about partners of sex addicts developing cancer from the emotional stress and trauma and I could feel why that would happen.

I was diagnosed with a boggy liver and told I had PTSD. I needed to do a better job of taking care of myself. I was told I couldn't workout at all other than walks and therapeutic yoga. Once again, I turned to my food. I knew that meat was tough on the liver (and alcohol, but there was no way in hell I was giving up wine at that time!). So I decided to go vegan to try and ease some of the burden on my liver and give my body more of the foods and nutrients it needed to support me through this time.

I had gotten down to 99lbs and I was sick constantly. Sinus infections, strep, skin infections, earaches, respiratory infections. I couldn't stay well.

I still hadn't made a decision about what to do. I wanted to leave. I felt like I had endured 14 years of a less than joyful marriage and now I understood why, and I had good reason to leave. But I also had counselors and friends saying things like…"Don't endure all of the bad and then miss the best he has to offer when he heals." "Do you want someone else to get the good version of him after you suffered the worst?" "What about the boys?"

This continued on for almost 9 months. Until one morning, we were all in the kitchen. Heath and I were standing on one side of the island and Jake was standing across from us putting syrup on his gluten-free, vegan pancakes. I was watching him when Heath reached over and put his hand on my shoulder. Without thinking I cringed at his touch and pulled away. And in that moment, I caught Jake's eye and I saw him react to my reaction.

And I knew. Right then…in my gut. I had to leave.

I was staying for my boys, but was that really serving them? This was the model I was showing them of a "loving relationship"? I suddenly realized that it would be so much better for them to experience two healthy, loving parents apart than two miserable, unhappy parents together. And I knew deep down that the co-dependent nature of our marriage meant that neither of us would ever properly heal as long as we were together.

It took me a few months to get up the courage to tell him and the courage to move forward without any answers as to how I'd survive as a single mom.

But somehow, deep down in my gut. I just knew it was the right decision and that being ok...well it was a choice. I'd do whatever it took.

I didn't want to be someone who survived her life. I wanted to be someone who thrived in life and that's who I became! Plants and how I ate weren't my only tools, but they were a huge part of my overall healing journey and prepared me physically and mentally to endure the stress, emotions, trauma and healing journey I experienced.

I'm not a doctor. I'm not going to quote statistics or use scare tactics to convince you to put plants on your plate. But I am going to tell you that in my personal experience, plants have power. Without them, I wouldn't and couldn't be the vibrant, youthful, joyful woman I am today. If my story and our recipes can help just one person thrive in life then this story, the book and all this journey is worth it to me. When we turn our pain into purpose, we can find joy in even the most intense struggles.

You are likely to come up with a lot of excuses about why eating more plants is too hard, too boring, too expensive and whatever else you need to tell yourself to justify not doing it. But I can tell you that I've had every one of your excuses and then some to not do it. And if I can do it, so can you! You don't need a lot of time. You don't need a lot of money. You don't need any fancy kitchen gadgets or special skills. You just need to have a desire to feel better and enough discipline to give it a fair shot. Like everything in life...it's a choice. What will you choose?

In just three years, I went from a woman who weighed 99 lbs suffering with PTSD who had no home, no job and no idea how she was going to take care of herself and her two boys. A woman filled with fear and insecurity. A woman embarrassed of the life she had allowed for so many years.

To a confident, healthy, strong, independent woman living out her dreams, serving others and choosing joy every day. A woman who believed in the power to create her own reality. A woman who didn't just survive but thrived. And I'm still going...this is just the beginning!

Your life could be dramatically different in as little as 12 months. Things are always changing. We just have to decide who's driving the change. Are you going to create a life you love...or live the life you're given by others? The choice is always yours to make.

If you'd like to learn about more of the tools I used on my transformation journey you can visit our blog at www.candnwellness.com and look for Calie's Tools For Transformation.

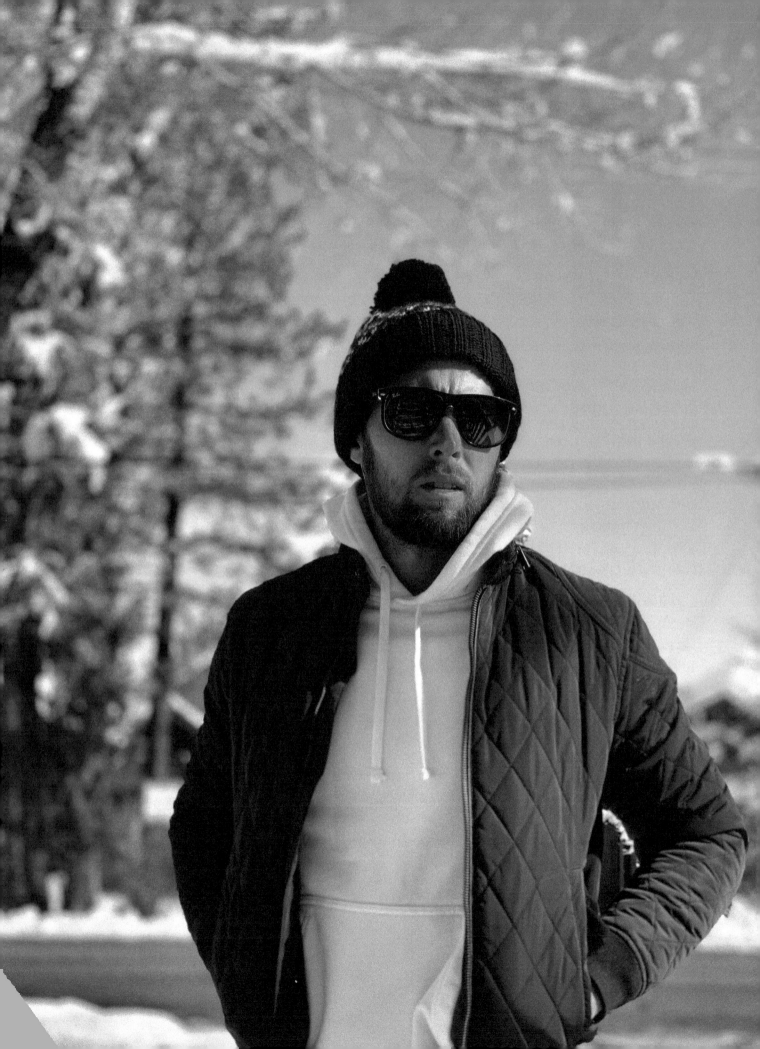

NIC'S JOURNEY

So, before sharing my journey with you, I better give an insight as to why I decided to collaborate with Calie on this book. It took a little persuading from her as I am actually a very private person. I have a very small circle of friends in my life (quality over quantity), I never really had any personal social media platforms and I don't read or watch the news. So this is a big step for me, but an exciting one. Calie said my story would resonate with some of you and could even be of help. So here I am, sharing my story. (I do have social media now as Calie said it will be a good idea to continue trying to help those who would like a more rounded, healthy lifestyle and could learn from my story). And as much as I am reluctant to it, that is the way the world is now so why not! One thing you will notice about me in this book is that I am very blunt and honest. You will also notice a few swear words so I just wanted to prepare you now!

Before you listen to me ramble on, and I mean this in the best way, I really don't care if you change your diet or become 'plant based' or 'vegan'. I will never tell someone to do something. I am just going to share my story of how I went from a lager drinking, fast food loving, suppressive boy, to a more rounded, health conscious man, who is trying to become a better person every day.

> **I am just going to share my story of how I went from a lager drinking, fast food loving, suppressive boy, to a more rounded, health conscious man, who is trying to become a better person every day.**

Childhood

I better start with my childhood because I am pretty sure most kids in England (and probably America) went through a similar one. I grew up in a seaside town Brighton, England. It is actually a really nice place to live, if you don't mind the rain! My focus was soccer and that's all I wanted to do. Lived, breathed and slept soccer (literally went to bed some nights hugging a soccer ball like an idiot). My mum and dad always gave me what I needed, and we were just your typical English family. Now, looking back from a nutritional standpoint, it was appalling. From the ages of 12 to 16, my diet was typical of a young English schoolboy. I would wake up around 7, spread a shit ton of butter and peanut butter (sometimes Marmite, which is like a black goo) on toast and pair it with a cup of tea which contained two heaped teaspoons of sugar. I would also just swig some milk out the carton and put it back. I never remember drinking that much water. I would annoyingly hurry my mum and sisters up so I could get to school early, so me and the boys could kick the ball around. I wouldn't eat again until around 12 which was school lunch time. My mum and dad used to put credit on one of those school café cards every Monday and that would need to last me until Friday. Every lunch, without fail would be a chicken burger (processed chicken), or a beef burger (don't even know what they put in that), fries and a can of Coke. Again, the only time I remember drinking water was if I walked past a drinking fountain so I would swipe a few sips. I would eat lunch as I was walking to the grass field so me and the boys could have a game of soccer before the bell rang. School would get out at 3, my mum would pick us up and as soon as I got home, I would stick on cartoons (Rugrats or The Simpsons) and chow down on the worlds biggest bowl of chocolate cereal. I would probably go out on the street and play more soccer or ride my bike before my mum would call me in for dinner. My mum, bless her heart, wasn't exactly the best cook in the world (luckily, she is now engaged to a chef), so she would just throw some food in the oven. A typical weekly dinner menu would consist of chicken nuggets and chips (fries), sausage and mash, corn beef hash (which I loved by the way), burger, chips and beans and maybe a small side salad at some point. Sometimes she would out do herself and make a Shepherd's Pie or Lasagna.

A typical weekly dinner menu would consist of chicken nuggets and chips (fries), sausage and mash, corn beef hash (which I loved by the way), burger, chips and beans and maybe a small side salad at some point

On Sunday's it would be your typical Sunday Roast dinner in England so that's where my mom had to do more than throw a few frozen foods in the oven. To be fair, her roasts were bloody brilliant. I think my dad would cook the chicken or beef because growing up "that was the man's job". Oh and without fail, after every dinner, me and my sisters would say halfway through, "what's for pudding (dessert)". We would either have a chocolate biscuit, ice cream, ice lolly or maybe a yogurt or something. But we ALWAYS had pudding.

Now, I don't blame my parents at all. They provided me with great meals, and I was never hungry. But they never took nutrition seriously because it wasn't really a priority. I don't even think it was a normal thing to do back then. The weekly shop that my mum did was planned out but not from a nutritional point of view. It was more of what we were going to have that week for dinner. As a kid,

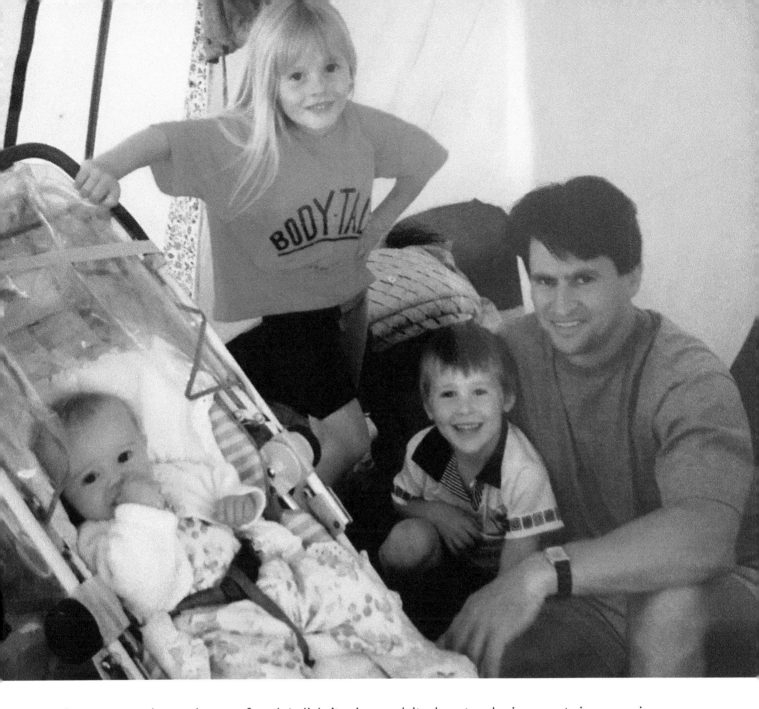

I just wanted good tasty food. I didn't give a shit about calories, protein, veggies or any of that stuff. Does it taste nice and will it fill me up were my only two concerns. I have asked my English friends if they had similar childhoods in terms of nutrition, and they confirmed it was pretty much exactly the same. Looking back, my parents weren't educated on nutrition, they just followed the same way they were taught by their parents.

Teenager 17

When I got a little older, around 17, I started to drink alcohol. I bought a fake ID and me and my friends would try and get into bars and clubs. My earliest memories of drinking started on Friday evenings. I used to tell my parents I was sleeping over at a friend's, but we would go buy a few liter bottles of vodka and take them to the local park. I recently asked my mum if she ever knew and she said "of course I bloody knew, I was the one who had to deal with your moody hangover the next day". We would spend hours there, just drinking having fun. I remember thinking it was one of the best times ever and I always looked forward to Fridays. Those Friday nights soon turned into Thursday Nights, Friday Nights and Saturday Nights. Because I was young, and everyone else was doing it, not once did I ever think of the negatives (apart from the raging hangovers). I played soccer at a pretty good level on the weekends so when I did wake up, I would take so Advil, down a can of coke, eat an English fry up and that would sort me out for the day. Once soccer was finished, it was tradition for the team to have a few cold pints together in the club house, have some sort of fried or fast food, and then head out that night to the clubs. This went on pretty much every weekend from 17 to 21. Looking back, I genuinely can't remember how much water I would drink. If I did drink water, it would usually be flavored. I would say my teenage years were filled with a lot of fun. A little too much fun to be honest.

My two childhood friends, Wai and Tom were always with me during the party phase and they were also on two completely different journeys. Wai was and

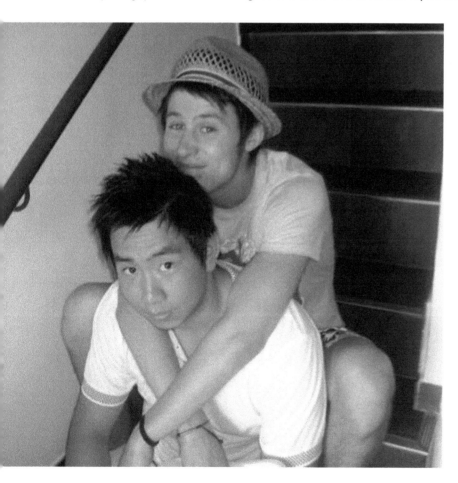

is one of the hardest workers I have ever met. He has been working since the age of 12 and even though he partied with us, his first priority was always work, and becoming more educated, more of a rounded person. I learnt so much from him and continue to do so. Tom had a different teenage journey too. He smoked, drank and got into trouble with the law. He always used to hang out with the wrong crowd and we kind of stopped hanging out because of it. I was afraid he would end up in jail. But if you look at him now, he is happily married, is plant-based Iron Man participant and is such a smart, humble and caring man.

College

At the age of 21, I moved to America where I was offered a soccer scholarship. I played in Montana and it was an amazing 4-year experience which I will forever be grateful for. Because I was on the soccer team, we had an eating schedule where the team would go to the canteen together and pick whatever we wanted (it was kind of a buffet style set up). I was team captain, in pretty good shape, but I also had the mental discipline of a 10-year-old when it came to food. Instead of going to the salad bar, I would be swayed towards tater tots, a burger, steak and fries. I would throw on a carrot or two because I could then lie to myself and say, "I am eating healthy". Oh and I would still wash all this down with a pint of Coke or a pint of Powerade. No one questioned it because everyone was doing the exact same thing. Even when our coaches would harp on about "eating healthy", we would all be thinking "fuck that, I can't wait for a burger". A running joke throughout the team was how I was always injured. And looking back now, I would always miss a few games every season. I know exactly why! I ate like shit, drank too many beers and didn't give a fuck what I was doing to my body. Because I was young and still looked good in the mirror, I continued doing what I have always done. It was also fascinating watching the younger college students around me party. Because of the drinking age in America, it seemed that these students could finally 'go nuts' and enjoy partying because they were no longer living with their parents. During my time at college, this was actually the first true sign my body was giving me that I ignored. Sophomore year I was outside Best Buy and had an appendix attack! Fucking painful. My mate took me to the hospital, and they had to surgically remove it. The doctors said I needed to make sure I maintained a healthier die.. Did I listen to the doctors or my body? Of course I didn't. Then comes Junior year. I was living with really sharp stomach pains for about a year. They would come on suddenly and I would have to go on my hands and knees and breathe heavily. Sometimes I would even stick my fingers down my throat to be sick as it would make the pain go away! I finally dragged my stubborn arse to the doctors and they said I had stomach ulcers. Yay, another procedure. I still have the images from the inside of my stomach. It's pretty gross as you can see where I was bleeding internally. So, after two surgeries in two years, and after graduating college, I would obviously change

> No one questioned it because everyone was doing the exact same thing. Even when our coaches would harp on about "eating healthy", we would all be thinking "fuck that, I can't wait for a burger".

my eating and drinking habits. Of course, I didn't!! I continued doing the same thing. Destroying my body. But everyone else was doing the same thing, so why change it!

Oregon

After graduating college, in 2013 I moved to Oregon. I started with absolutely nothing. Literally a loaf of bread in the cupboard and a few cans of pasta. I worked as a soccer coach and built my way up and started my own business. I had a really good time in Oregon and met some brilliant people, but this is where my life started to take a downwards turn. My eating and drinking habits remained the same. I would get on with my day and go off to work like everyone. But every evening I would have a drink or two. That was my "relaxing time". My "I deserve this cold beer" time. I never thought I was doing anything wrong. But one or two drinks a night, plus more on the weekend, that's not healthy at all! Alcohol was also a way I dealt with my problems. You know after a long day or something negative has happened, you get home and say to yourself "I need a drink." Driving home after something pissed me off in my day, I would get excited about getting home and cracking open a cold one. I would pour myself a Moscow mule or a beer, and those first few sips were amazing. I would forget my problems and focus on the exciting things happening in my life. Halfway through the drink that initial buzz would slowly fade, and I would start thinking about that problem at work, my relationship or whatever it was. So, I would pour another and get that buzz back. My eating habits were just as bad. I would wake up and have toast with butter, lunch I would buy fast food (usually two McChicken Sandwiches from McDonalds and a coke) and for dinner, I would either stick some fries and a burger in the oven (just like my mum did for me growing up) or I would go pick up some Chinese or something. Because I went to the gym every day (just doing heavy weights) and also joined in with soccer whilst I was coaching the kids, I thought I could balance it all and still feel good.

In 2016/2017, this was the time where everything came crashing down really. I felt completely lost, I had no drive and I didn't really know what the fuck I was doing. I felt like a robot.

In 2016/2017, this was the time where everything came crashing down really. I felt completely lost, I had no drive and I didn't really know what the fuck I was doing. I felt like a robot. It is easy now to see what I did wrong, but at the time I hadn't a clue. I thought I was just going through a bad period in my life and I couldn't control it. The only time I felt myself and happy was when I was at home, enjoying a cold pint and watching a movie with my dog. It was my escape from my problems. I always put on my mask when going to work, pretending I was happy and making sure the kids I were coaching were having a good training session and were having fun. Because I was so stubborn, and didn't want to confide in anyone, I hid my problems well from everyone. Sometimes I would go home and cry, sometimes I would go home and be angry and other times I would just sit at a bar, having a couple of beers. Mentally, I was fragile and upset. But as a typical man, I hid it. My body wasn't getting what it needed both physically and emotionally. I started to let little things really bother me, and it effected my business. I wasn't the same guy anymore. I let so many people down. I always knew the kids would be fine, youth soccer is just that, youth soccer. They would continue without me or

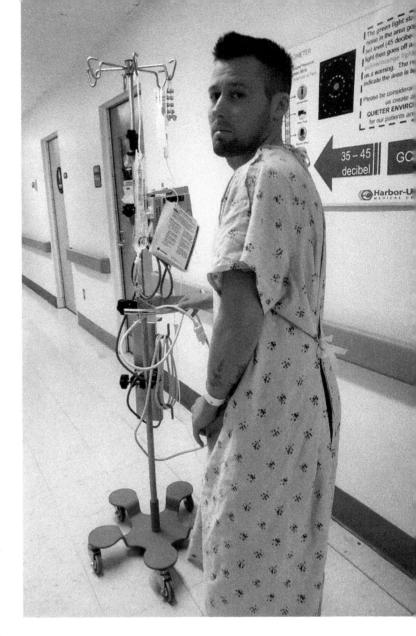

find another team. But it was the people who put time and energy into me and my business that I was disappointed about. One of my closest friends was a guy called Mark. He was there at the beginning and at the end and I thought of him as an older brother. A sweet guy who always wanted the best for those around him, including me. He was hilarious and we had tons of fun together.

Everything seemed to get on top of me. Whenever a problem occurred, instead of dealing with it with a call to action type of attitude, trying to figure it out, I was in the mental state of "fuck it, I'm not dealing with that". Now that I understand energy and what your mental and physical state have on your day to day life, of course problems kept on finding their way to me. It got so bad; I ran away from them. I literally packed up all my shit and moved and I didn't tell anyone. I made up excuses, and just left Oregon. Of course, there are two sides to every story. The backlash was horrific and there were so many lies I had to listen to created by the people I left. But I created the problems in the first place. I was selfish, angry,

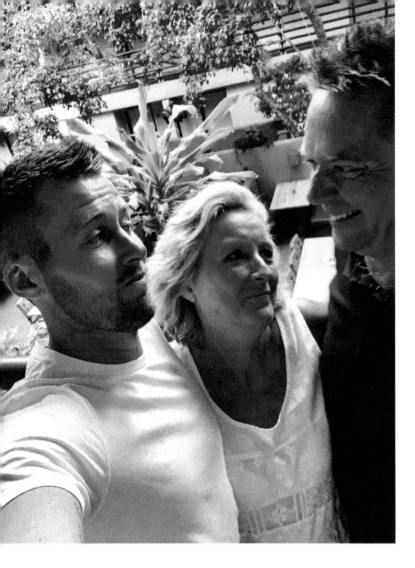

lost and genuinely didn't know what direction to turn in. To this day, I will always miss the youth soccer players I coached, I had some amazing relationships with them and hope all of them are reaching their potential and enjoying their lives. During this time, my relationship with my family back in England completely collapsed. I was still close with my dad, but even he was extremely worried about me.

When I moved away from Oregon, I remember struggling to breathe at times, so I went to the doctors. The doctor gave me the typical response which I think they are just trained to do...."you are depressed, take these anti-depression drugs" and sent me on my way. I have never really taken any prescription drugs apart from when going through surgeries, so this was a little blow to me and my pride.

I remember sitting in my apartment looking at the bottle and being so angry at myself! These pills won't change anything, maybe short term, but they are just a bandage, covering a wound. I need to deal with my problems internally, myself. Not with prescription drugs or alcohol. Both were just an excuse to justify needing them. So I made the decision to start understanding why I felt the way I did and I threw those pills in the trash. In the space of a year, I moved to New Mexico and to California. When I moved to California in June 2017, I was a 29-year-old who could fit all of his life into his car. That was pretty sad.

California

During my first year in California, I continued to have a few beers at the weekends and eat like shit. I signed up to the dating apps and continued just going through the motions. A great friend of mine, Ricky, told me that I suppressed my feelings a lot. No one ever said that to me before, and it really hit home. I did. Every time something "bad" happened or I faced a problem, I would laugh it off or deal with it by having a beer and pretend it was all fine. He would always make sure I was on the right track and helped as much as he could. But how do you help someone who thinks they didn't need help? Fair play to him, he stuck with me. To this day we are very good friends and I owe it to him for getting my shit together and getting back at it.

I felt like I was just about starting to get my life back on the right path and I started to feel like myself again. I would only have one or two beers on the weekends, I started eating healthier and I had a great job coaching in soccer again. I was lucky enough to work with some great coaches and the kids would always make me smile during training and on game days. Watching kids grow on and off the soccer field is really a great experience for a coach and one that I will always enjoy. I typically live my life by quietly learning from people. Understanding the strengths and weaknesses of those around me and taking them on board to try to make myself better. I was surrounded by really good people in Los Angeles, so I was constantly learning. I lost a lot of passion for soccer during the end of my time in Oregon, but I met a guy who helped me fall in love with the game again. Paul is a Director at a soccer club and his passion for the game and to help soccer players develop really opened my eyes again to what passion meant. One stand out person who gave me a different outlook was a friend of mine called Sonia. She is an extremely hard-working person. Always putting the needs of others first before herself. She is honest, genuine, and very caring. People like Sonia you want to keep in your circle! So if you have someone you know like her, my advice is to keep them with you!

So in typical Nic fashion, what did I do...I spent the next two weeks suppressing my feelings. Pretending everything was okay.

Suddenly, life decided to throw me a problem. On my Birthday, my dog died. That was a kick in the arse. He was a good little dog. I picked him up from the shelter in Oregon in 2014 and he went everywhere with me. He was only 4 when he passed. He got hit by a car. So in typical Nic fashion, what did I do...I spent the next two weeks suppressing my feelings. Pretending everything was okay.

A few months later, the day after Christmas Day, my dad died. My dad was a good man. Always kind and always put the needs of others first. Sometimes maybe too much! He was quiet and serious most of the time, but he had a goofy side to him as well which I loved. My dad and I would Facetime a lot when I moved to America and he always wanted to make sure I was doing alright. Because of the time difference, he would usually call around 10pm England time. This is when he would be in his kitchen, enjoying a few beers and a Brandy. As much as I loved our chats, my dad was always either buzzed or drunk when we would talk

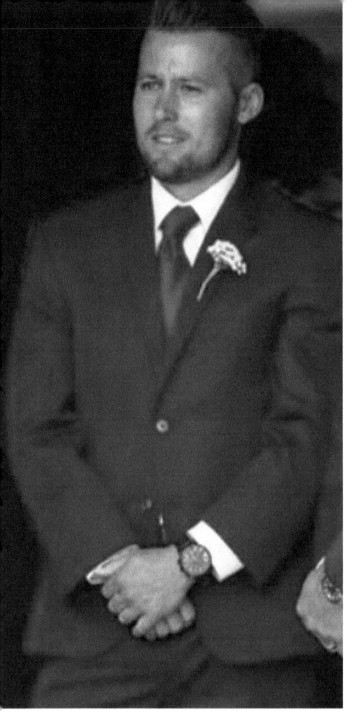

on the weekends. I knew he had a drinking problem and would often tell him. But it fell on death ears. I was worried about him. He was also a suppresser. I could see the pain and sadness in his eyes when we spoke, but he always said everything was fine. And I always said I was fine. So you have a father and son, both suppressing our feelings and never talking about them to each other. He would ask me what was wrong, and I would ask him. It was like a tennis match but with no winner. Looking back now, I really wished I asked him more questions and I also wish I opened up to him. By doing that, maybe he would have opened up to me. My dad is one of the biggest reasons why I have changed the way I behave, what I put into my body and how I now open up to people close to me about my feelings. I owe my dad so much, and that is why I dedicated this book to him.

I actually met Calie a few days after my dad passed (we will go into this a little more in the next section "OUR STORY"). During 2018, I started to reconnect with my mum back home in England. I started to get my life back on track again. Everything was going well. But I still suppressed my feelings about my family, about how I left Oregon and my feelings and emotions regarding my dad.

Hospital

Since the appendix surgery and the ulcer surgery, I still lived with an excruciating pain in my stomach. Every month or so for the past 5 years, I had stabbing stomach pains. Because they occurred once a month, I just dealt with the pain and didn't go to the doctors. Not once did I ever think "is it because I'm drinking alcohol, is it because I'm not eating healthy meals". Of course I didn't. I dealt with it.

I was watching How to Train A Dragon 3 with my girlfriend at the time. My once-a-month stomach pains started to happen at the start of the movie. I rubbed on my stomach which always helped contain it, but for some reason it didn't this time. I went outside and walked around the block. Continuously for an hour trying to stop the pain. Once the movie finished, my girlfriend came out and we drove to hers. About 1am, my pains were still horrific, so I do phase two of "How Nic deals with pain". This was to have a hot bath. I remember being in the bath, on my hands and knees because the pain was so bad. I didn't sleep a wink that night. When my girlfriend woke up, the pain told my stubbornness to fuck off and get my ars to urgent care. We went to a small Urgent Care in LA and the doctor took my temperature...104!

Part of me didn't want to
be expensive! But again,
choice. When I checked
Close to passing out!
finally kicked in and
told me I had HUGE gall
I that I have had them
the years of stomach
then be transferred to
Torrance. Well most of you
so laying in an ambulance
great time. Anyway, because it

During this time, I used it to write some changes I wanted to make. There is something freeing about writing your problems down.

She told me to get my ars to hospital.
because I knew it was going to
my body didn't give me a
into hospital, I was in agony.
My new friend Morphine
I was relaxed! The doctors
stones. Golf ball size and
for years (that explains
pains then). I had to
a specialized hospital in
probably know LA traffic
during rush hour wasn't a
was the weekend, the surgical team

wouldn't be in until Monday, so I had to just wait. I was hooked up to an IV and every four hours they gave me pain meds. I wasn't allowed to eat which was the worst part!

Monday was surgery day and they were going to remove the gall bladder. Everything went well and I was recovering. They put a stint in me (I think to help drain stuff) I don't actually know because I was out of it on pain meds. I was excited on Wednesday morning because I could eat again! I hadn't had anything to eat since Friday evening at the movies. I had some jello and the world's worst tasting soup. A few hours went past and then boom...I had a pain that I could only describe as ten people stabbing me. I was on my hands and knees on the hospital bed, covered in sweat. The nurse and doctor were giving me ice to cool me down, but I was in agony.

I was rushed down to the MRI room and they said the stint had gone into my pancreas. I was sent down for another two surgeries and recovered for the remaining week. This was the official start of my new journey.

It took a few weeks of doing nothing to Recover. During this time, I used it to write some changes I wanted to make. There is something freeing about writing your problems down. It was like my mind finally being able to unload and talk to me. I of course cried as I was writing my lists. I was really annoyed at myself

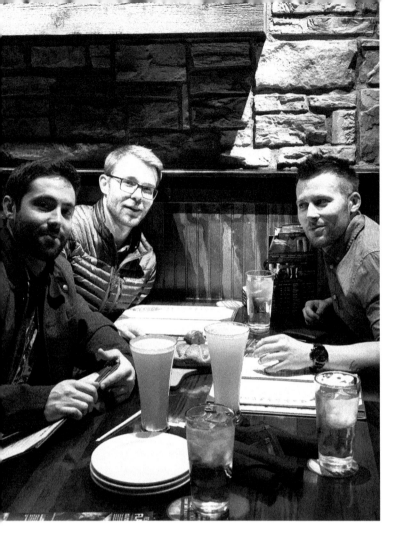

for how the past 2 years went. People always say, "you have to let go of the past". I get that, but I couldn't help but look at how much of a dickhead I was. I listened to nobody and did whatever I wanted to do, with no thought of the consequences. I wrote how much I typically drank on a weekly basis. Even one pint of beer or cocktail in an evening, a few days a week isn't healthy. But I justified it somehow. I also wrote what I wanted to achieve in life. This list after my 'near death' experience, was to be the start of what I see now as "NEW NIC".

The next few months went by and I started to get healthier. Less shit food and less alcohol. I still had some heavy nights though on the weekends! Which is crazy to think about now for someone who was still recovering from surgery. I decided I wanted to build a house in memory of my dad, so I moved back to New Mexico on June 1st, 2019 and started work on it. The weeks went by, and I was starting to feel myself again. But there was still a niggle at the back of my mind, and I didn't know what it was. And in typical Nic style, I just ignored it. July 23rd will forever stand out like a sore thumb. This was the day, for some reason, my mind literally told me to stop doing what I was doing. I needed to really start listening and make some solid changes.

I am not religious in anyway, and I was never spiritual. I am the type of person who must see something to believe it. Still, I cannot tell you why on July 23rd something changed inside. But I started to take notice. But really take notice. I let my ego go and decided to write another list. But this time it was going to be a completely honest list. Not a list that deep down I knew was actually me lying to myself. But an honest list.

I closed my eyes and pictured what I do day to day and how I act. I pictured what my mind thinks about and what excites me. Well, the truth is, it was still the same things as the past 13 or so years of my life. Working hard and playing hard. I would get really excited about finishing a good week of work at the house, and then going out with friends and having a few pints. I then thought about what I feel like the morning after. Guilt, anxiety, feeling of letting myself down all came to mind. My dad would pop into my head to and I could feel myself letting him down. After writing out a huge list, I decided to put it into practice. Why do I get annoyed, why do I drink, what problems am I facing right now and how can I deal with them etc etc. The list went on and on. I started to think about my past relationships and how I was still single and why. I started to think about all my visits to hospital and why I still don't feel healthy. I started to think about my career and why I still had a void. Once I answered these questions honestly, it gave me a new sense of direction. I was going to be disciplined and stick to it.

Plant-Based

The main priority was health. So, after watching documentaries, reading books and listening to a close friend of mine, Brianna, I decided to really change my eating habits. So, I thought I would try to stop eating meat. I, Nic, the guy who loves a rare steak, boneless chicken wings and a meaty burger, was no longer going to eat meat. And because I like to challenge myself, I thought why not go the whole way. Just become a plant-based eater. I didn't have social media or read the news, but I had a good understanding of how "Vegan" or "plant based" eaters were viewed to others. I didn't give a shit about that because I was doing it for myself and my health. I also prepared myself for my friends' comments once I told them. And right on cue, the sly laughing came, the "why" questions came, and I could feel them almost looking at me like I was some kind of alien. Again, I really don't care what people think about me, never have done, but it was really interesting to see people's reactions. Especially when you go against 'the norm'. I am currently 9 months into my plant-based journey. Along the way, I have researched it more and more and figured out which foods I like and honestly, which foods taste like shit. For example, I bought a chorizo plant-based sausage, cooked it at home and it tasted like a shoe. The point is, not everyone will like the recipes in this book, but finding the foods you do like, and putting your own spin on them will help.

Of course, I do feel good knowing I won't be eating another animal, helping the worlds carbon footprint and all that good stuff. But in all honesty, if this plant-based diet didn't make me feel good, I would go back to meat. But, I have never, in my 32 years, felt better. As I walk around grocery stores, of course I look down at a massive steak and my mouth waters, but I now have more respect for the animal itself and won't touch the little guy.

Alcohol

I have completely reigned in my drinking habits. I will have the occasional beer but honestly, I no longer get the same cravings as I once did. Especially to go out and 'party'. Instead of going home and cracking open a cold can of beer, I crack open a cold sparkling water. I also set myself a rule. If I do have a drink, it will be in a social environment. I won't drink on my own. Another rule is to pace my drink. Usually, that cold beer or fruity cocktail would be in my belly within ten minutes. By the time I was halfway through, I already knew my next drink decision. Now, I take as long as possible to drink my first one, and if I fancy a second, I will have it. But typically, that would be it.

I definitely see the world differently now. Situations and people that used to annoy me, no longer do.

So basically after my rambling, if someone asked me a before and after summary, this is what I would say.

Before July 23rd, 2019

- My body gave me more than enough signs during my life to say, "STOP and CHANGE". I treated my body like shit.
- I watched my dad drink a lot, and he passed away. I also watch my close friends drink way too much (and my family). So it worries me.
- I thought about how it felt when being buzzed or drunk. I hated waking up the next morning and feeling like shit!
- My energy levels whilst eating meat and not having a balanced diet declined
- My skin kept breaking out
- I saw how negative I became. Getting annoyed at silly things.

After July 23rd, 2019

- I work out once a day (cardio and weights)
- I only have a drink in a social environment (typically a few times a month)
- I changed my diet. I now only eat plant-based. My energy levels have increased dramatically, my skin feels great and physically my body is in good shape.
- I read, I meditate, I manifest, I give gratitude. All these things have helped me see the world completely differently. I have also distanced myself from negative situations (unfortunately this has meant losing some friendships).

I definitely see the world differently now. Situations and people that used to annoy me, no longer do. Instead of blaming ex-girlfriends for the break down in relationships, I acknowledge what I could have done better and learn from it. Instead of scrolling through pointless YouTube videos, I read. Instead of jamming out to loud music on the way to work, I listen to podcasts from guru's, philosophers, or educators. Instead of eating fast food, I cook and meal prep. Instead of hanging out with people that are negative or not on my current path, I distance myself from them. Instead of eating meat and dairy, I eat plant-based. Instead of drinking alcohol every day or even a few times a week, I drink water. Since changing my habits, I honestly have never felt better. I am happy, I am healthy, and I am positive.

I do have some very open-minded people around me though. They are in my corner. One of whom I have met recently, Selacia. She is a writer, DNA intuitive healer, spiritual teacher and someone I am extremely lucky to know. She doesn't deliver bullshit, or a therapy session. She is in tune with the universe and someone who I trust to help guide me and answer questions I have along the way. If you are into this type of spiritual guidance, or even just a little intrigued, I would highly recommend finding someone like Selacia. (Even mentioning this is crazy to me because if someone told me I would be speaking to a spiritual guide a year ago, I would have told them they are talking nonsense).

> **Another big part of my journey has been the people that have come and gone. I have had some close friends that have drifted apart.**

Everyone is different, but if I was to give someone advice based on my own changes, it would be this;

1. Being honest with YOURSELF. Acknowledging that you have a problem/s.
2. Understanding what you can do about them the natural way. Not by taking all the prescription chemical stuff.
3. Putting a plan together to achieve the changes you want.
4. Maintain a disciplined routine to make sure you reach your goals of change!
5. No excuses, no bullshit. If you want to change, change. If you don't, that's down to you.

Moving Forward

I wrote this outlay of my life in January 2020. I wrote it over a space of a few weeks, coming back to it from time to time, adding a few things. But like I said before, my hope is that if my story resonates with someone, that will be brilliant. Looking back at my life, it is easy now to see the mistakes I made. I had surgeries because I treated my body like shit. My business in Oregon collapsed because I wasn't giving my mental state any honest time or thought. My relationships broke down because I didn't communicate my feelings.

Another big part of my journey has been the people that have come and gone. I have had some close friends that have drifted apart. I have realized now that it isn't personal, we are just going on separate paths at the moment. One of the most important lessons I have learnt during this journey is that you do have to be honest with yourself and stay on a positive frequency. I have some friends that party too much, take anti-depressants and pain killers, hate their jobs, are not happy in their relationships or situation. And I have found that when you surround yourself in that environment, it is easy to be drawn back into it and I found myself doing just that. So I had to again, make a difficult decision and distance myself from some close friends. That isn't me saying " I'm better than them". It just means I need to go on my own path for a while. I do honestly hope one day our paths cross again and we can reconnect. I will always wish my friends a happy and healthy life.

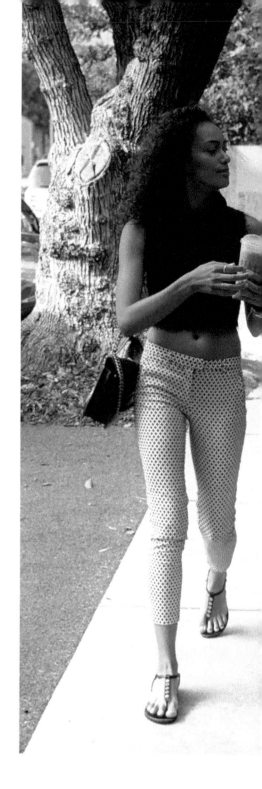

It has also been fascinating watching those close to me shift their habits. The two people I least expected was my mum and her fiancé, Eric. They came to visit me in America in September 2019. It was the first time I have seen my mum since we fell out back in 2016. My mum said she immediately saw a difference in my energy and positivity. She said "you are not my son" in a jokey way. The next 10 days were brilliant. I shared my stories with them and the journey I am on. What I didn't expect was them to show real interest and ask to learn more. We had long discussions during our trip, how we view the world, diets, drinking habits etc. When they returned to England, they had a plan to change their normal routine and wanted a better, more healthy life for themselves. It has been a slow start, but it is their start. That's all that matters. They have already made strides and I can already tell a huge difference.

My best mate Wai is now on a similar journey to me. I share my stories with him, I share quotes and videos from guru's and philosophers, and we have some great Facetime talks on how we now see the world. Because Wai works long hours (he is a very successful multiple business owner) he shares his struggles with me on how its hard for him to continue a plant-based diet whilst always travelling for

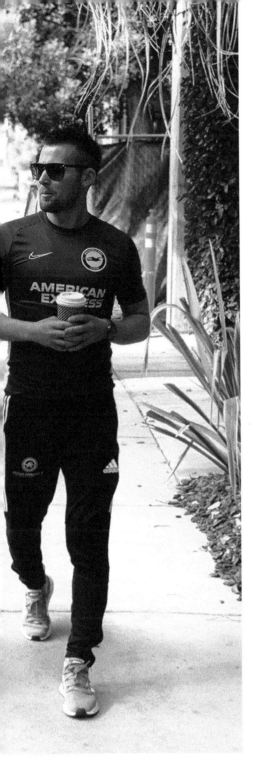

work. He knows that it is just an excuse, he openly admits that, so we come up with ideas on how he can maintain a plant-based diet whilst continuing to live his busy life.

My childhood mate Tom has entered multiple Iron Man events, continues to eat only plant based and he said how much it has helped him with his extreme training. He says his energy is so much higher than when he trained whilst eating meat.

My other two best mates, Brianna and Ricky, are on the same journey and we speak every day. Brianna as mentioned previously, is the one responsible for me and Ricky becoming plant-based. She models all over the world and maintains a plant-based diet. She has had a troubled past like most of us have, but is always full of energy and positivity. Watching her grow into her career has been truly great to see.

Ricky is a successful businessman who has also rapidly changed his eating habits. Ricky has always been a healthy eater and loves going to the gym. But he has suffered some painful injuries and they used to creep up on him from time to time. Since his change to plant-based, along with maintain a positive energy, he is extremely happy.

My 2020 goals are to remain disciplined in my lifestyle. To make sure I am grounded, honest and positive with everyone and everything I do. I will continue to eat right, only drink occasionally and socially and to make sure the people in my circle are looked after. Life is exciting and is there to be lived, it's just a matter of finding out what YOU want to do with it.

After the "Journey" sections of this book, the following recipes are a guide for those who don't really know too much about a plant-based diet and also for people who are open to try some. Calie and I have rated the recipes and you will notice that some of them one of us loves, and the other think tastes like shit! But that's the whole point. No one likes the same food all the time.

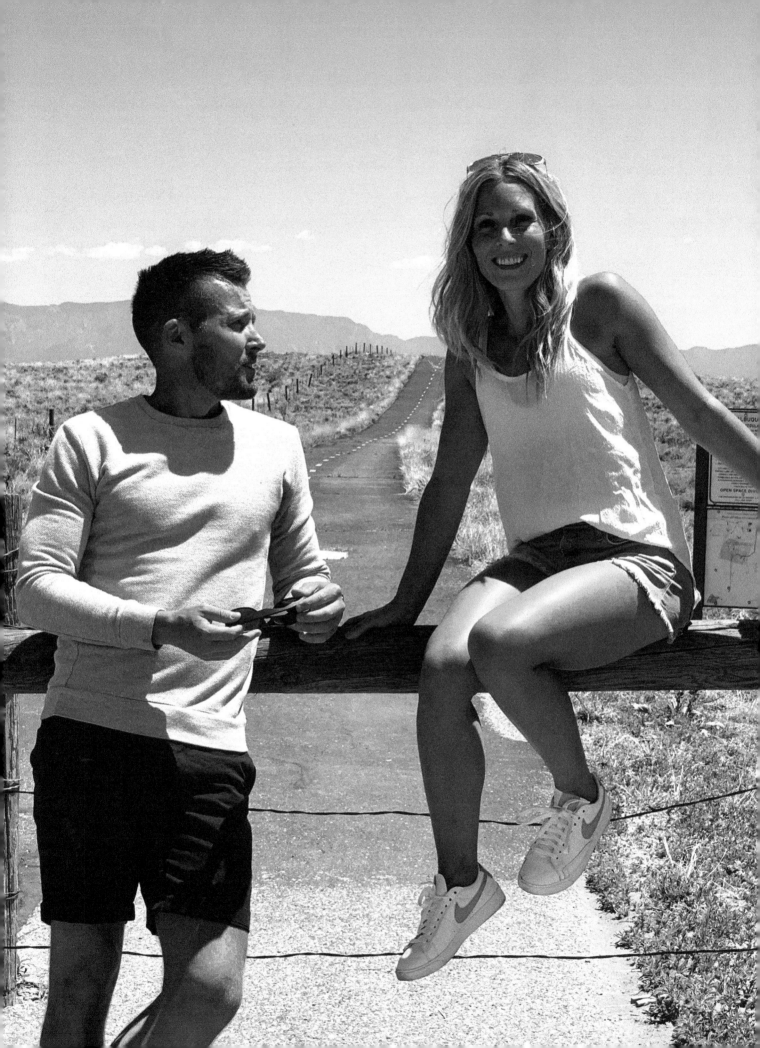

OUR JOURNEY

We met at a time when neither of us really should have been dating. Nic had just lost his Dad and Calie was still recovering from a traumatic divorce. But things always happen for a reason. Which was something Nic frequently reminded Calie of...especially whenever she would ask about their relationship.

Nic and Calie...we were actually a ton of fun together. We laughed a lot. We ate a lot of great food. We drank...a lot! We took impromptu road trips. We shopped together...we both love shopping! We did boring routine stuff too.

Together, just the two of us. We were really good. Or so it seemed. But the truth was. We were both still healing. Both still hiding. Both still needing to do a lot of work on ourselves, so our relationship....well it was pretty superficial.

Despite all the texts and calls and time we spent together we never talked about anything real. We didn't really share our feelings...ever. We didn't talk about our futures, our struggles, our stories. We put on our happy faces and tried to be who we thought the other person needed and wanted us to be.

> Nic and Calie... we were actually a ton of fun together. We laughed a lot. We ate a lot of great food. We drank...a lot!

Of course...neither of us was remotely aware of that fact at the time.

Calie was still working hard to get back on her feet after the divorce and was trying to grow her social media following post 80 Day Obsession along with her Beachbody business. Nic was also working hard to get back on his feet, coaching and starting a new business.

Calie started to realize she wasn't being herself around Nic. She always pretended everything was great, but frequently cried when he wasn't around out of stress and financial fear. She never asked for what she really wanted and pretended not to be disappointed when she didn't get it. Nic wasn't aware of any of this at

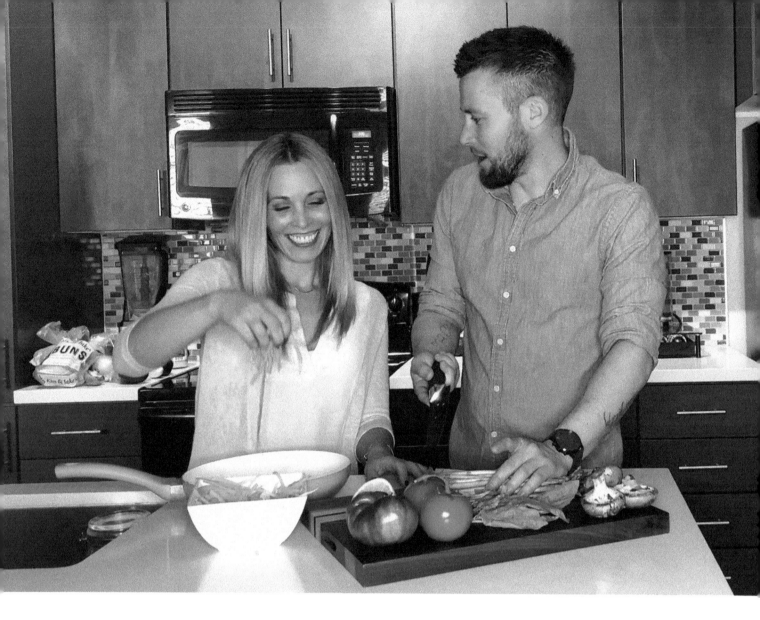

the time. He knew Calie was still going through a tough time, but when asked her if she was okay, she always said she was.

Calie's thoughts were swirling out of control and she didn't know what to do. But she knew that she was quickly falling into unhealthy habits and losing herself and her voice in this relationship. She also knew it wasn't Nic's fault. She had worked hard to gain her independence and she wasn't willing to lose it. But she wasn't strong enough to tell him that.

He called later that night and she promised herself she'd discuss it with him. And she didn't. Nic was going about his usual business, picking up groceries for the night after practice. Calie was into her third glass of wine and crafting a text to tell Nic all the things that she didn't have the courage to actually say to him.

Calie hit send and waited. The phone didn't ring. No text came through. She drank another glass of wine. Still nothing. She cried.

The next day Nic replied...disappointed and done. Because of the struggles he faced over the last two years, he was still in an angry state of mind. Always thinking people were dickheads. He took the text as a breakup and that was the end of Calie and Nic. No "let's talk about this". And following the same pattern as he did in Oregon, he just thought "fuck it".

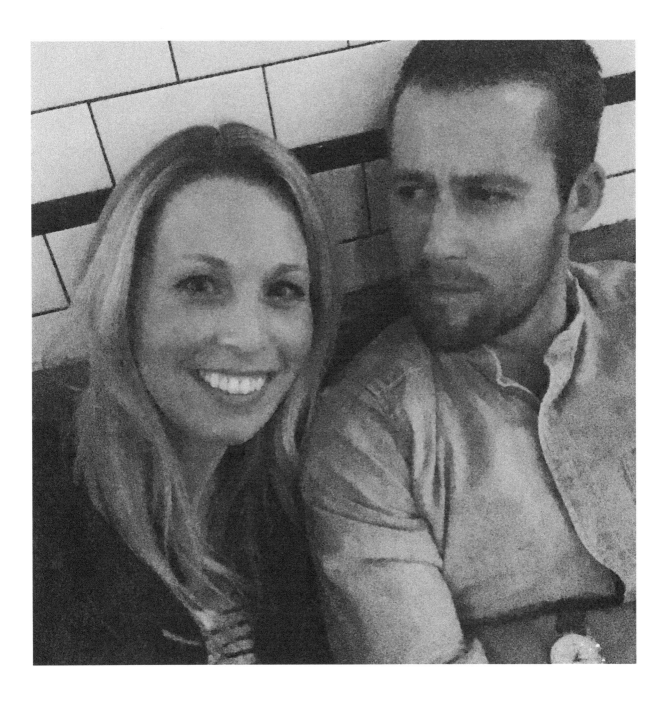

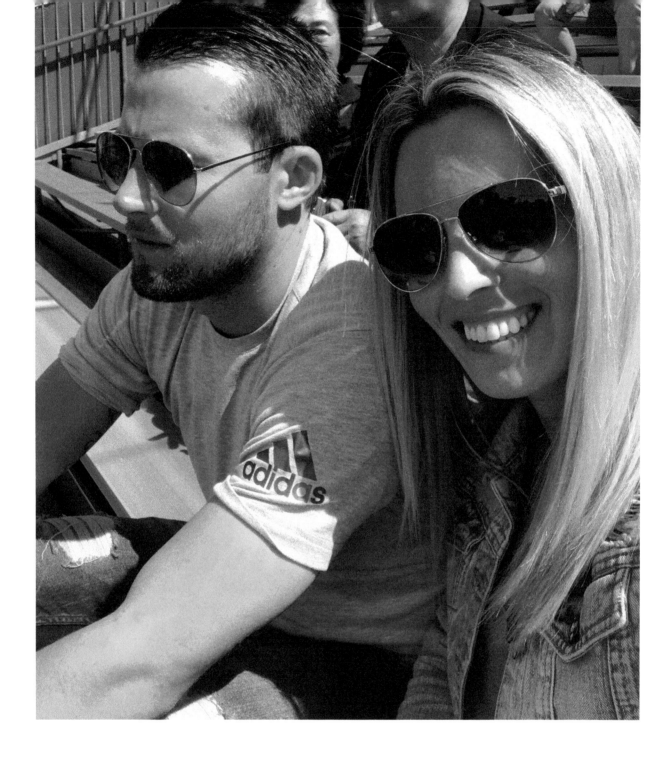

Three months later, Calie reached out to Nic and asked if he'd be willing to meet for coffee. They met at a coffee shop and actually had a great conversation. It was surprisingly comfortable...or so Calie thought. Afterward, she sent a text saying how great it was to see him and suggesting they keep in touch as friends.

Nic didn't believe in being friends with exes and that's exactly what he told her. Watching his parents divorce and his friends relationships breaking down around him, he had the stigma attached to it. "There is no need to be friends with an ex".

He then Followed announced that he was planning to move to Albuquerque. And that was the end of Calie and Nic.

Nic eventually moved to Albuquerque, bought a house and started working to remodel it. Calie moved on with her life, kept working on her personal development, took a 5 month hiatus from dating and focused on her boys and building her business.

We are grateful for everyone who picks up this book and shares their time with us. We hope that our stories and our recipes inspire you to explore your own health and healing journey.

They both had significant other relationships. They both hit new lows in their lives as part of their healing journeys. They both got into spiritual work, gratitude work, and creative visualization and manifesting. And they both got real honest with themselves and started making hard but necessary changes in their lives.

Calie and Nic reconnected via Bumble. He felt the need to reach out to Calie and he knew he would find her on there (for some reason he just knew). Low and behold, she was fifth in the line of women he saw. They talked and exchanged numbers. Sharing their new journeys with each other in such an honest and open way.

As you can probably assume...their friendship grew and over the course of the next few months...the idea for Plant Based...Well Kind Of was born out of the similarities in their journeys and the hope that their individual stories could help others just like them to live healthier, happier lives.

We are grateful for everyone who picks up this book and shares their time with us. We hope that our stories and our recipes inspire you to explore your own health and healing journey.

Our journeys are far from over and we continue to share them on our website where you can read more details and get ongoing support, recipe ideas and inspiration for living a more authentic, honest, vibrant life. Come visit us at www. candnwellness.com or follow us on Instagram @nicpheff and @coachcalie.

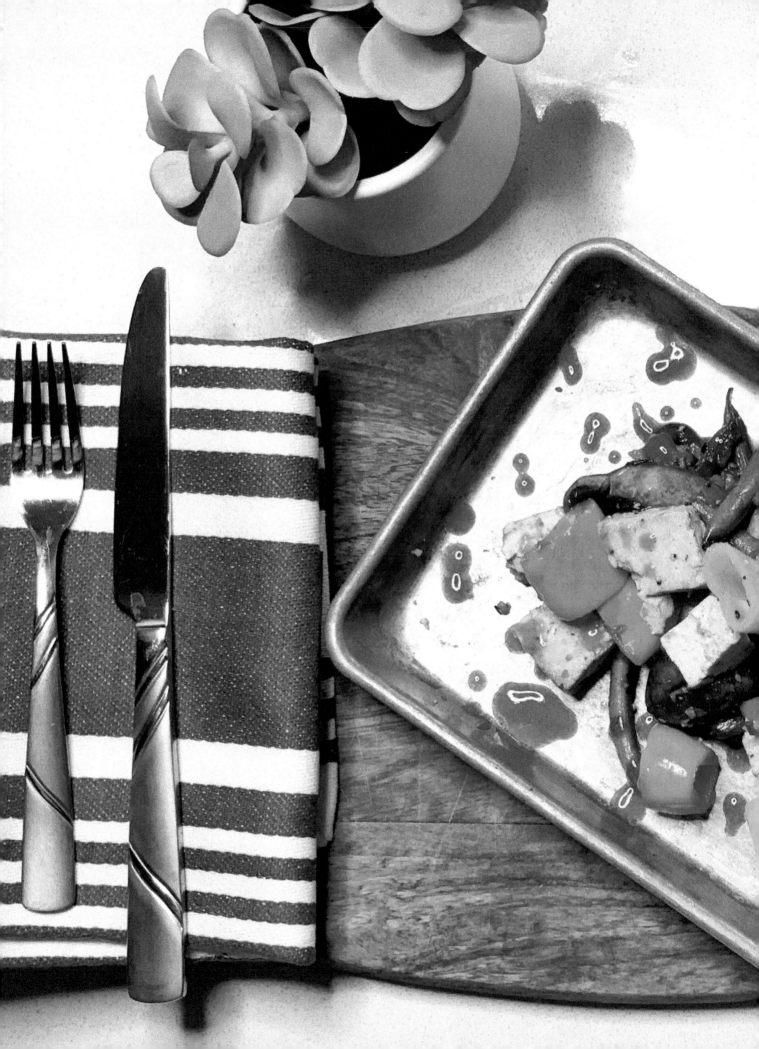

BREAKFAST

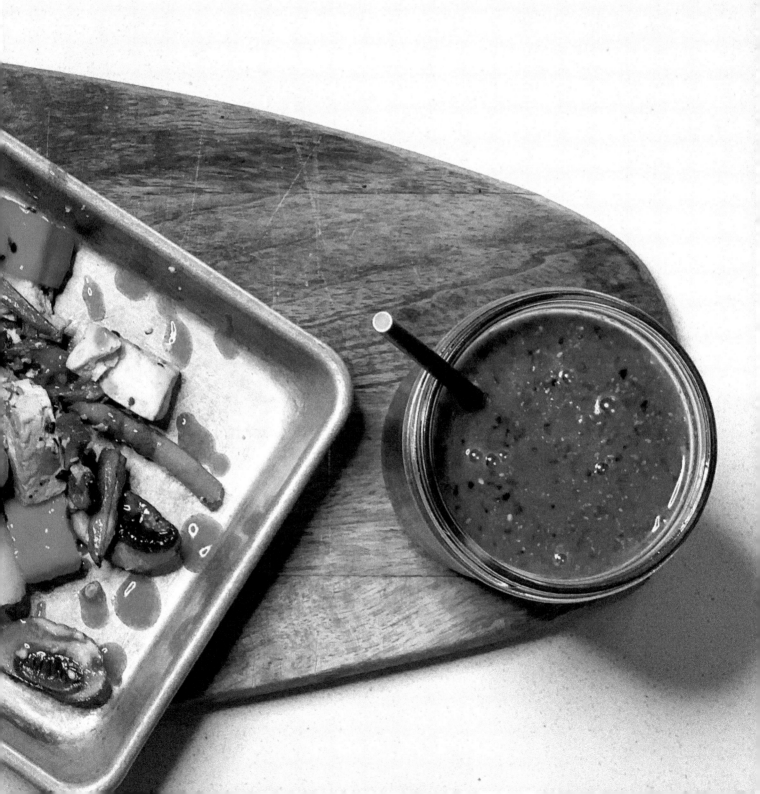

BREAKFAST

Superseed Smoothie

INGREDIENTS

We're giving you approximate measurements here so you can get a good smoothie consistency

- ¼ cup of acai juice
- ¼ cup of carrot juice
- A few splashes of aloe vera juice (pure, not other ingredients added)
- Handful of spinach
- ½ banana
- ½ cup of frozen mixed berries
- ½ cup of frozen cauliflower
- 2 Tablespoon of chia seeds
- Tablespoon of flax seeds
- 8-10 raw almonds
- Optional vegan protein powder

DIRECTIONS

Throw it all in a blender and blend until smooth. Easy!

OPTIONAL ADD INS

1. You can swap any of the juices for water or unsweetened almond, oat, or coconut milk
2. Switch up the fruits
3. Add cacao powder, vanilla extract or even maple extract

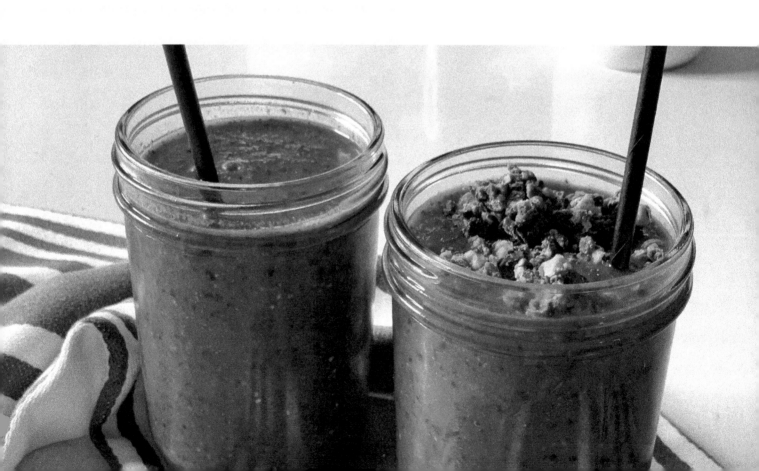

Pairings

alie - Fajita vegetables make a great topping with the avocado and some fresh cilantro

Nic - Buffalo Sauce

BREAKFAST

Avocado Toast

and remove it in a pretty photo worthy fashion. Add a few slices of tomato and sprinkle with salt, black pepper, and garlic powder. Squeeze a drizzle of lemon juice on top and bosh! 5 minutes to a delicious breakfast or snack.

OPTIONAL ADD INS

1. Change up the seasonings. Red pepper flakes, rosemary, onion powder...
2. Add fresh herbs. Basil is ridiculously good especially if you add some soft vegan cheese.
3. Throw on some plant-based protein like smoked tempeh, mashed garbanzo beans or cannellini beans.
4. Can't go wrong with superseeds like sesame seeds, pumpkin seeds, sunflower seeds.
5. Hit it with some spice...Sriracha, Cholula, or our favorite buffalo sauce.

INGREDIENTS

- 1-2 slices of bread of your choice. There are lots of vegan bread options out now. The healthiest options are usually in the freezer or cooler section. Calie uses gluten-free/vegan bread. Nic eats 2 slices and Calie would eat 1.
- Vegan butter (We both love Earth Balance Original.)
- Avocado
- Cherry tomatoes
- Salt
- Black pepper
- Garlic powder
- Lemon

DIRECTIONS

Toast your bread. Spread some butter on it. Top with avocado slices or just mashed avocado if you can't be bothered to slice

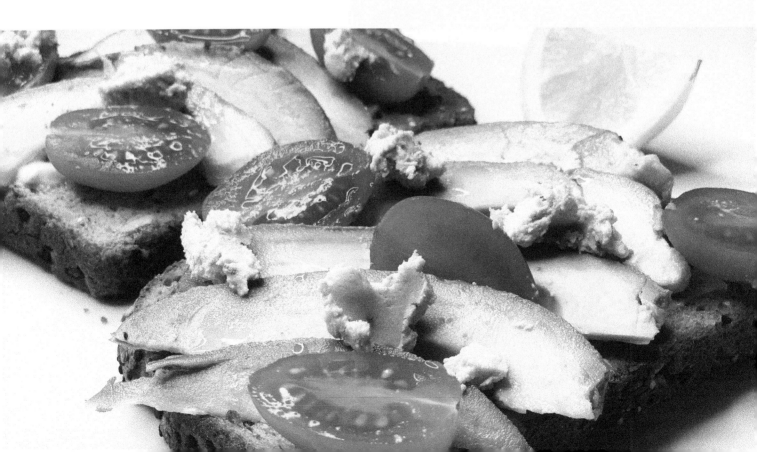

BREAKFAST

Garbanzo Toast

INGREDIENTS

- 2 slices of whole grain vegan bread
- ½ box of garbanzo beans
- hummus
- Cherry tomatoes
- Lemon
- Salt
- Black pepper
- Olive oil

DIRECTIONS

Toast your bread (obviously and if you don't have a toaster 1. Just get one and 2. You can also toast your bread in the oven or in a skillet with a little vegan butter.

You can literally just spoon the garbanzo beans right out of the box or can (no fucking excuses), but it does taste even better if you make just a tiny bit of effort and warm them in a pan with olive oil.

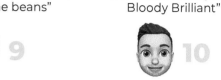

Spread the hummus on your toasted bread. Top with your cold or hot garbanzo beans, add a few slices of cherry tomatoes, drizzle with lemon juice and sprinkle with salt and pepper.

*At the time of writing Nic is literally eating this every morning for breakfast and it keeps him full until noon.

OPTIONAL ADD INS

1. Herbs guys...do we need to keep writing it?
2. Any seasonings you like. Red pepper flakes, chili powder, cumin, paprika...now my mouth is watering again.
3. Change the bean...black beans, white beans, use what you got!
4. Hot sauce....always hot sauce!

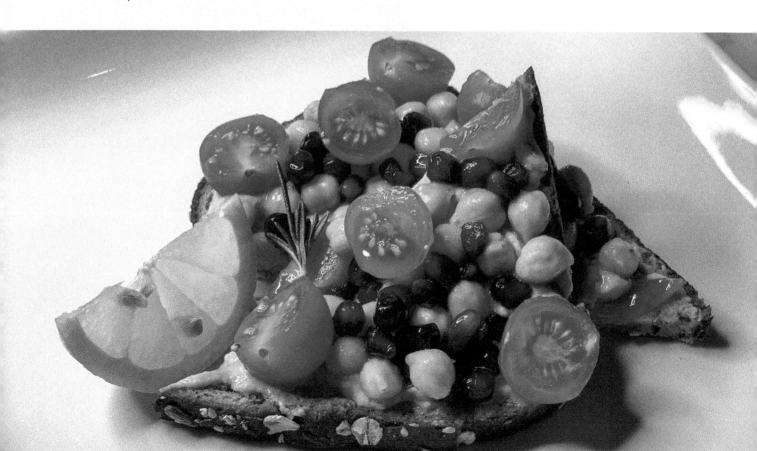

Ratings

Calie - "This is how start most days and it makes me feel amazing!"

 9

Nic - "Good veggie intake to start the day"

 7

Pairings

Calie - Buffalo Sauce

Nic – As is

stirring occasionally. Taste test for flavor and add additional seasoning if needed.

Remove from heat and serve.

OPTIONAL ADD INS

1. Add organic sprouted tofu cubes. Use extra firm. Press the tofu between two plates to drain excess water. Cut into bite size cubes and add to the pan for 2-3 minutes before tossing in your veggies.
2. Sprinkle with 1 Tablespoon of hemp hearts after plated for a boost of plant based energy and protein.
3. Calie loves to toss in a Trader Joe's HI-protein veggie burger before the veggies. Break it up as it cooks into crumbles for a great pop of flavor and protein. This makes it more filling and is one of Calie's go to pre-workout meals.

BREAKFAST

Vegetable Medley

INGREDIENTS

- Handful of asparagus - chopped into bite size pieces
- Handful of diced bell peppers - red and yellow
- Handful of sliced baby bella mushrooms
- Drizzle of olive oil
- Salt to taste
- Trader Joe's Everything But the Bagel Seasoning to taste
  - Substitute - Sprinkle of garlic powder, onion powder and sesame seeds

DIRECTIONS

In a small skillet, drizzle olive oil and heat over medium. Toss in all of your veggies and sprinkle in your seasonings. Mix well to coat with oil and spices. Cook for approximately 10-12 minutes

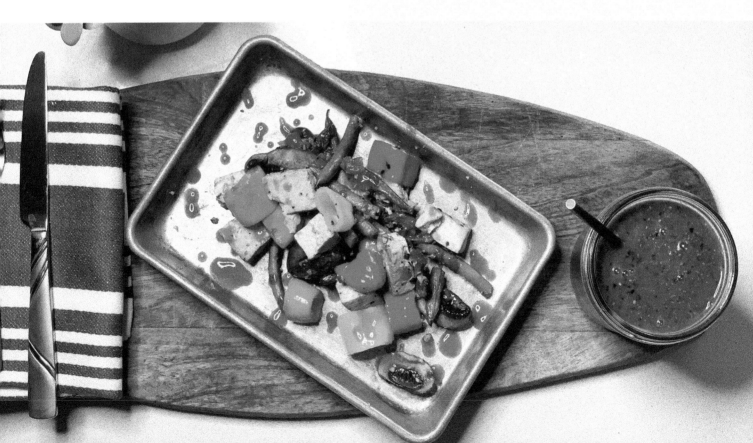

BREAKFAST

Grain-Free Granola

INGREDIENTS

- 1 12 oz bag of raw organic cashews (chopped)
- Small handful of roasted and unsalted sunflower seeds
- Small handful of organic pumpkin seeds
- 2 Tablespoons-ish of chia seeds
- 2 Tablespoons-ish of banana flour (substitute almond meal if you can't find banana flour)
- 2 Tablespoons-ish of unsweetened shredded coconut
- Heaping ⅓ cup of peanut butter (I love Santa Cruz...no shitty peanut butters you see on commercials loaded with sugars and fillings and preservatives...your body hates it! I promise.)
- 2 tsp of unrefined organic coconut oil
- About 2 teaspoons or a little more of pure maple syrup (again, not the fake crap! Splurge for the real deal and just use a little.)
- Sprinkle of cinnamon
- Few dashes of Salt

DIRECTIONS

Toss all of the ingredients in a bowl and mix it with your hands. It helps melt the coconut oil and peanut butter and ensures everything coated evenly for the best flavor. Get a little messy. It's fun. A food processor will turn it into creamy butter, which might taste good but not what we're going for here.

Preheat the oven to 325 and spread your granola on a baking sheet lined with parchment paper. Bake for approximately 20 minutes stirring half way through. Let it cool then store it in a jar with a lid. Good for a week but won't last that long!

OPTIONAL ADD INS

1. You can use any unsweetened nutbutter instead of peanut butter in the same ratio.
2. Feel free to sub the cashews for pecans, almonds or walnuts. Walnuts are a little more bitter flavor but still work if you enjoy them.
3. Add other spices like nutmeg or even cacao powder or cacao nibs after it's cooked and cooled

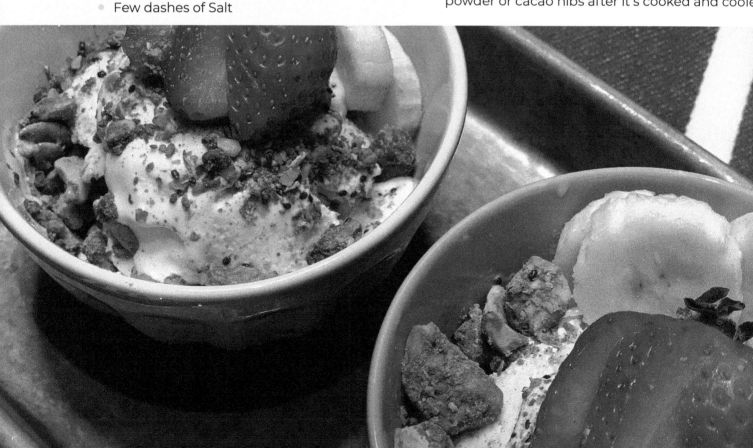

Prepare your flax egg. 1 Tablespoon of Flax seeds + 2.5 Tablespoons of water per egg. Mix it well with a fork and let it for 2-3 minutes before adding to your squash.

Sprinkle in some cinnamon and drizzle in a little maple extract maple syrup and blend well.

In small skillet, greased with a little coconut oil, pour about cup of pancake mix into the pan and cook just like a pancake.

Top with your favorite toppings. So many options! You never have to eat the same pancakes twice.

OPTIONAL ADD INS

You can also try substituting a really ripe banana mashed for the flax eggs. It's sweeter and a little thicker, but still really delicious!

You can use ½ cup of pancake batter and make them thinner then use as a wrap for sunbutter and mashed berries. Kind of like a crepe!

Change up the toppings. Sautéed plantains are a really great compliment to the butternut squash.

Make a savory pancake by changing up the toppings. Squash, maple and sage go really well together. You can top with sage and fennel infused lentils or sautéed greens and smoky tempeh for an indulgent and filling Sunday morning brunch.

BREAKFAST

Butternut Squash Pancakes

INGREDIENTS

- 1 cup steamed cubed butternut squash
- 2 flax eggs (non-vegans you can use eggs)
- Cinnamon
- Maple extract or pure maple syrup (just a drizzle)
- Toppings of your choice - we used blueberries, dried cranberries, almonds, maca powder, unsweetened coconut flakes and unsweetened sunbutter drizzle
- Coconut oil

DIRECTIONS

If from frozen squash:

Steam your butternut squash. You can use the microwave if you're pressed for time, but honestly, it kind of ruins the health benefits. I just toss it in a pan with a few tablespoons of water over medium heat and put a lid on it so it steams. Cook until you can easily mash it with a fork.

If from fresh squash:

Bake a butternut squash whole at 425 for about an hour. Cut it in half, scoop out the seeds then scoop out the squash. Use a cup of squash mash per serving. You can freeze the leftovers or make extra pancakes because these will be gone in minutes.

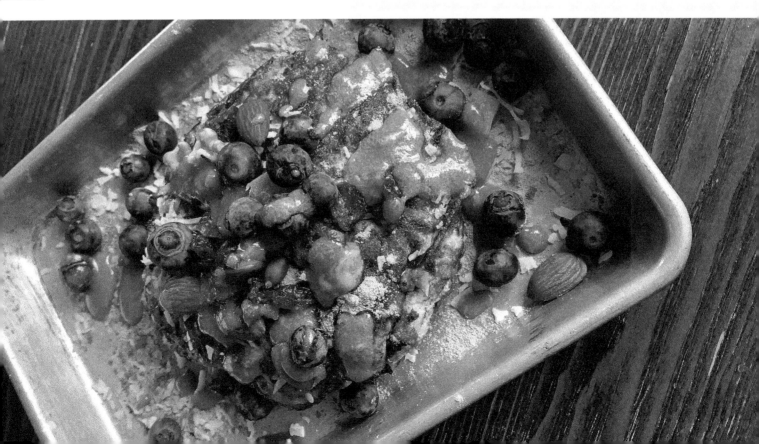

BREAKFAST

Coconut Yogurt Belly Bowl

INGREDIENTS

- Unsweetened coconut yogurt (we like a probiotic rich brand like Cocoyo)
- Variety of colored fruits you enjoy (we used raspberries, kiwi, pineapple and wild blueberries for this variation)
- Superfoods of your choosing (we went with hemp hearts, flax seeds and maca powder)
- Healthy fat (we used raw, organic walnuts)

DIRECTIONS

This is the easiest breakfast to make and it's so good for your gut. If you have the time, you can lay out in the bowl for a pretty presentation because we do eat with our eyes first and it makes a great Instagram post. But honestly, it's all going down the same way, so grab the ingredients of your choice, throw that shit in a bowl and mangia (that's Italian for eat!) Your body and belly will love it!

Ratings

Calie - "If I'm not starting the day with a veggie medley then I'm probably having this."

 8

Nic - "So good"

 9

Pairings

Calie - Kale chips because it's always good to get some morning veggies in

Nic – I'd have this with a bagel

OPTIONAL ADD INS

1. You can also use almond milk yogurt or any other non-dairy yogurt, but the coconut brands tend to have the most live probiotics for that healthy gut microbiome.
2. Any fruits will work - fresh or frozen. Try to minimize dried fruits because they're really higher in sugar and canned fruits are usually highly preserved and lose their nutritional value over time.
3. Mix and match your superfoods but you're looking for things like chia, hemp, flax, spirulina, maca, cacao powder and even cinnamon.
4. Any nuts or seeds or even unsweetened nutbutters.
5. You can also always add a little granola like our grain free granola for some crunch and texture.

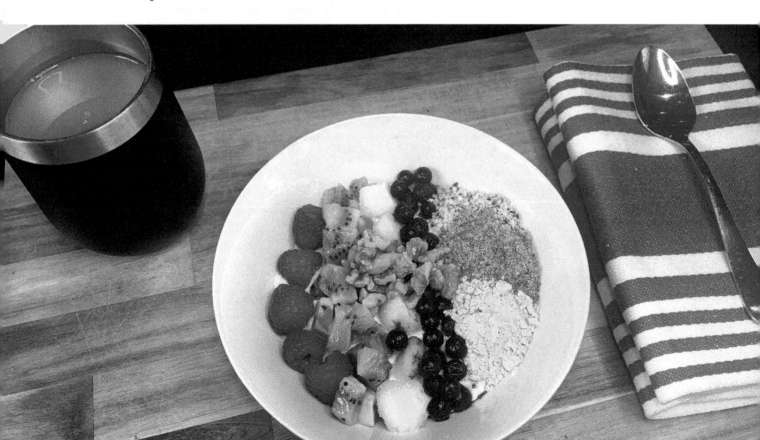

alie - "If I'm not starting the day with a veggie medley then I'm probably having this."

 8

Nic - "So good"

 9

BREAKFAST

Acai Bowl

INGREDIENTS

Just like the smoothie, we're giving you approximate measurements here so you can get a good consistency

- 1/2 cup of acai juice
- ¼ cup of almond milk
- Handful of spinach
- 1 Banana
- ½ cup of frozen mixed berries
- Handful of fresh blueberries
- ½ cup of frozen cauliflower
- Tablespoon of chia seeds
- Tablespoon of flax seeds
- Teaspoon of honey
- 8-10 raw cashews (or any nut of your choice)
- Optional vegan protein powder
- Optional Granola topping

DIRECTIONS

Throw it all in a blender but save half a banana, the blueberries, chia seeds and honey. Pour mix into bowl, put the slices of banana on top, along with the blueberries and chia seeds.

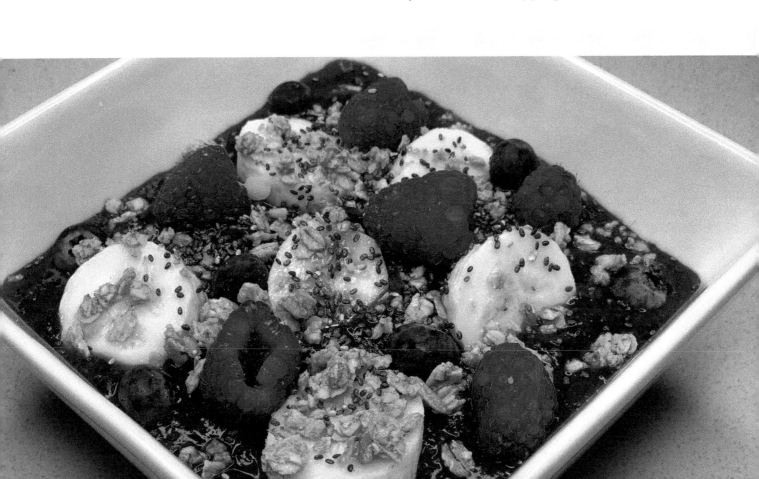

BREAKFAST

Banana Split

INGREDIENTS

- Banana (peeled, obviously guys)
- Maca powder
- Hemp hearts
- Goji berries
- Wild frozen blueberries
- Unsweetened almond butter (or whatever nut butter you like)

DIRECTIONS

Let's be honest, can you even call this a recipe? Just top your peeled and sliced banana with whatever superfoods make you happy. But here's what we did.

Drizzle a small spoonful of almond butter over the banana. Sprinkle with hemp hearts and maca powder (ladies, this is great for energy and libido...just sayin). Toss some goji berries on top and drop a handful of wild

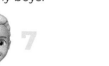
frozen blueberries on it because they basically have the highest antioxidant level around. SOOOO good for you!

OPTIONAL ADD INS

1. Any plant based superfood - flax seeds, chia seeds, cacao nibs...
2. Any chopped nuts or other seeds like walnuts, pumpkin seeds...
3. Any other fruit like raspberries, mulberries, cherries....

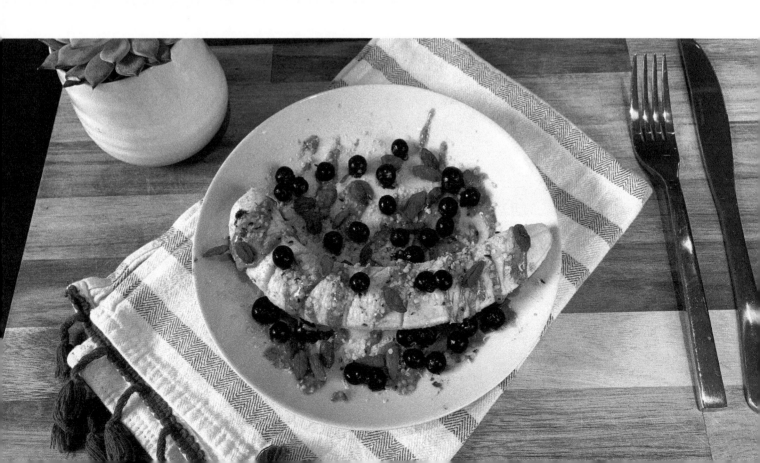

Ratings

Calie - "SOOOOOO GOOOOOD"

 10

Nic - "Fuck yes. Who wouldn't want pizza for breaky"

 10

Pairings

alie - This one is so filling. just eat it alone or pair it with some fresh berries.

Nic – As is

epper. Calie adds red pepper flakes because she likes verything spicy. (It's why her and Nic can be friends.) aste it as you go. The sage and fennel give it a "sausage" avor.

p with arugula, tomatoes, and mozzarella.

ake an additional 2-4 minutes to warm the toppings and nelt the cheese.

nd if you're like Calie, hit it with some hot sauce before erving!

PTIONAL ADD INS

You can use any vegan pizza crust or one of the grain free wraps that Calie and Nic used in their cook-off.

It's pizza so the toppings are endless. Mushrooms, onions, bell peppers, spinach, fennel...

Vegan parmesan cheese mixed with the mozzarella is really delicious.

If you are going for plant-based and not vegan Calie used to eat this with two runny eggs on top and old Nic would have added ground beef (but called it mince).

BREAKFAST

Breakfast Pizza

* Store bought vegan crusts are the easiest and most realistic. We rarely (ok, never) make our own crusts even though we could

- about ⅓ cup of cooked lentils
- arugula
- cherry tomatoes
- Miyokos mozzarella cheese
- Sage
- Oregano
- Garlic Powder
- Salt and black pepper
- Fresh Basil
- Olive oil
- Cholula hot sauce

DIRECTIONS

Preheat the oven according to your pizza crusts directions. We prefer the Cauli-Flour Foods gluten-free and vegan Italian pizza crust for this recipe. While the crust is cooking, follow the directions on the lentil bag to cook your soon to be "sausage" lentils.

When your crust comes out of the oven, drizzle it with olive oil and a little oregano for that pizza flavor.

Mix your lentils with a heaping sprinkle of sage & fennel, a little salt, garlic powder and black

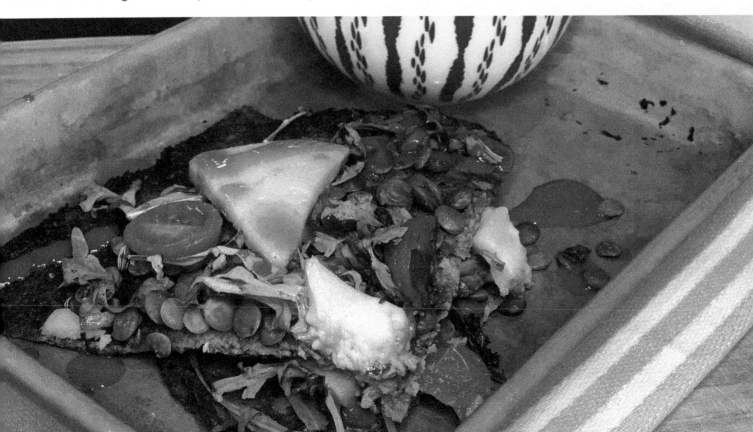

BREAKFAST

Berry Cream Cheese Bagel

INGREDIENTS

- Vegan bagel or vegan ezekiel english muffin (look for minimal ingredients and best found in the freezer section)
- Vegan cream cheese - we love Kite Hill's plain
- Small handful of fresh raspberries
- Blueberries
- Granola

DIRECTIONS

This is really just assembly. The only direction is to add ¾ of your fresh raspberries to your cream cheese and mash them until well blended. Then toast your bagel/english muffin. Spread your raspberry cream cheese on top. Add some fresh whole berries and sprinkle with a little granola.

OPTIONAL ADD INS

1. Any additional superfood seeds like chia, hemp hearts, or flax seeds
2. Sprinkle of maca powder for a little vanilla flavoring
3. Unsweetened coconut shreds
4. Drizzle of honey or almond butter

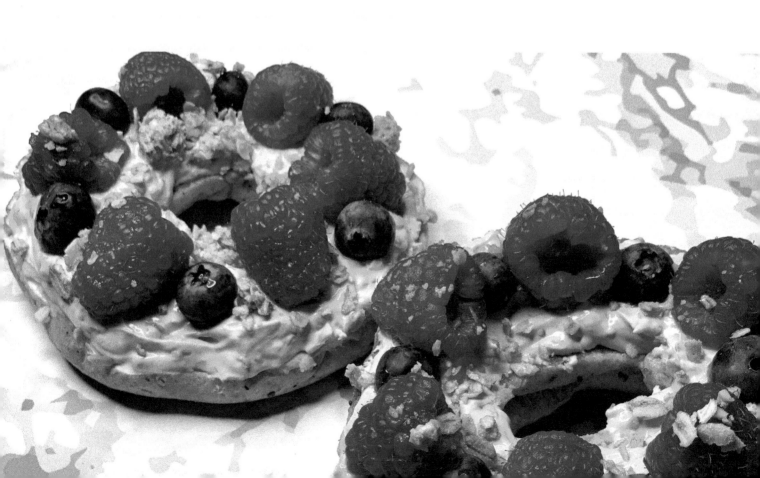

Cherry Pie Oats

Ratings

ie - "I love oats, but they
on't love me back. This
ne's for you guys. Trust
me...it's delicious."

9

Nic - "Never been a fan
of oatmeal"

4

Pairings

alie - Vegetable medley
½ serving

Nic - Granola

and cinnamon. It's so delicious! Creamy, sweet, filling. A great preworkout meal.

OPTIONAL ADD INS

1. Change the fruit and change the flavor.
2. Change the oats. There are so many options for hearty breakfast bowls like millet (more crunchy and nutty), farro (thicker and creamier), brown rice (heavier and takes on any flavor). Little swaps help you avoid boredom, keep it easy and provide more nutritional variety.
3. Crushed pecans are another favorite topping of ours.
4. You can always add superfoods like maca powder, chia seeds, flax seeds, etc.
5. Think of a pie flavor and add the appropriate fruit, crushed nuts and spices that you would use in that pie. Have fun with it!

INGREDIENTS

*I measure my oats to get the right consistency

- ½ cup of uncooked old fashioned rolled oats (I find these are easiest for most people to digest)
- 1 cup of water
- 8-10 frozen dark cherries
- Sprinkle of chopped walnuts
- Drizzle of pure maple syrup or maple extract
- Drizzle of unsweetened almond butter
- Dash of salt

DIRECTIONS

In a small pan, bring water with a dash of salt to a boil. Add your oats, stir, cover and simmer over low for about 10 minutes. Watch it closely because oatmeal is like avocados, it goes from perfect to ruined in a minute.

Spoon into a bowl and top with dark frozen cherries, nuts, nut butter, maple syrup or extract

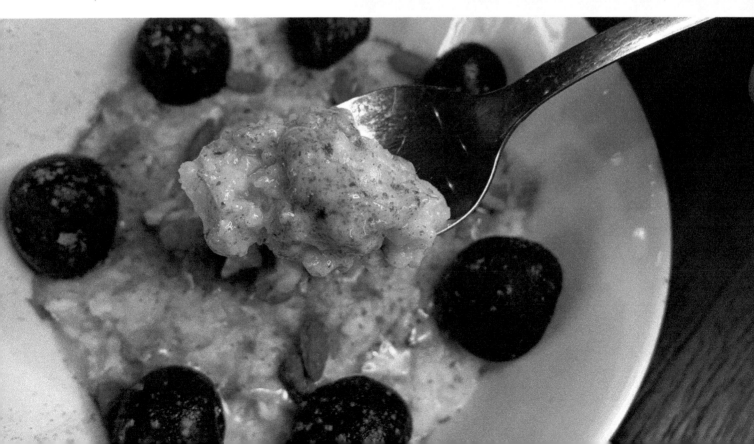

BREAKFAST

Sweet Potato Toast

INGREDIENTS

- 1 small sweet potato (Calie prefers purple sweet potatoes & Nic likes the traditional orange)
- Organic, unrefined coconut oil
- Hummus
- Spinach
- Tomato
- Salt
- Cumin
- Turmeric
- Black pepper

DIRECTIONS

Preheat your oven to 425. Cuts sweet potato ends off then slice into ¼ inch thick rounds. Spread a little bit of coconut oil on each side to keep them from drying out. Sprinkle with a little bit of cumin, turmeric, black pepper and salt. Spread onto a baking sheet and bake for about 25 minutes until soft in the center.

Top with hummus, spinach and tomato slices.

Ratings

Calie - "My weekend go to! Never gets boring."

 8

Nic - " Love a good sweet potato"

 8

Pairings

Calie - Balsamic mushrooms

Nic - Kale Chips

OPTIONAL ADD INS

1. Be creative. How would you top toast? Fresh herb like basil and rosemary add tons of flavor and extra nutrients.
2. Dice up some onion and mushrooms and sauté those bad boys in a little olive oil with salt and pepper. Put that on top of the humus for an extra hearty toast.
3. You can always add tempeh, veggie burger crumbles, hemp hearts, flax seeds or even an egg if you aren't vegan and are just cutting back on animal protein and increasing your plant intake.

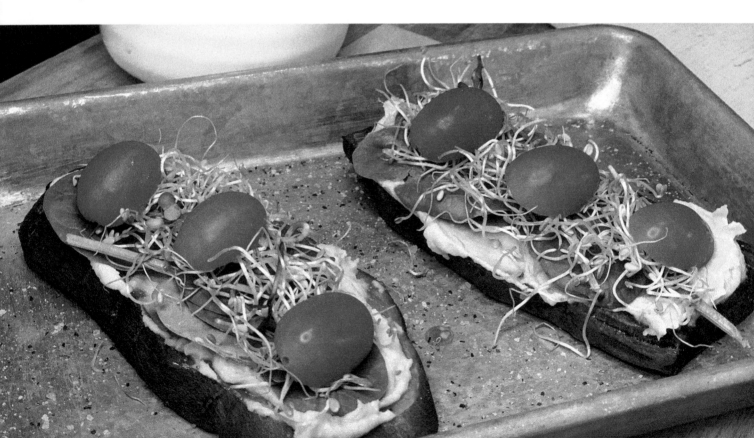

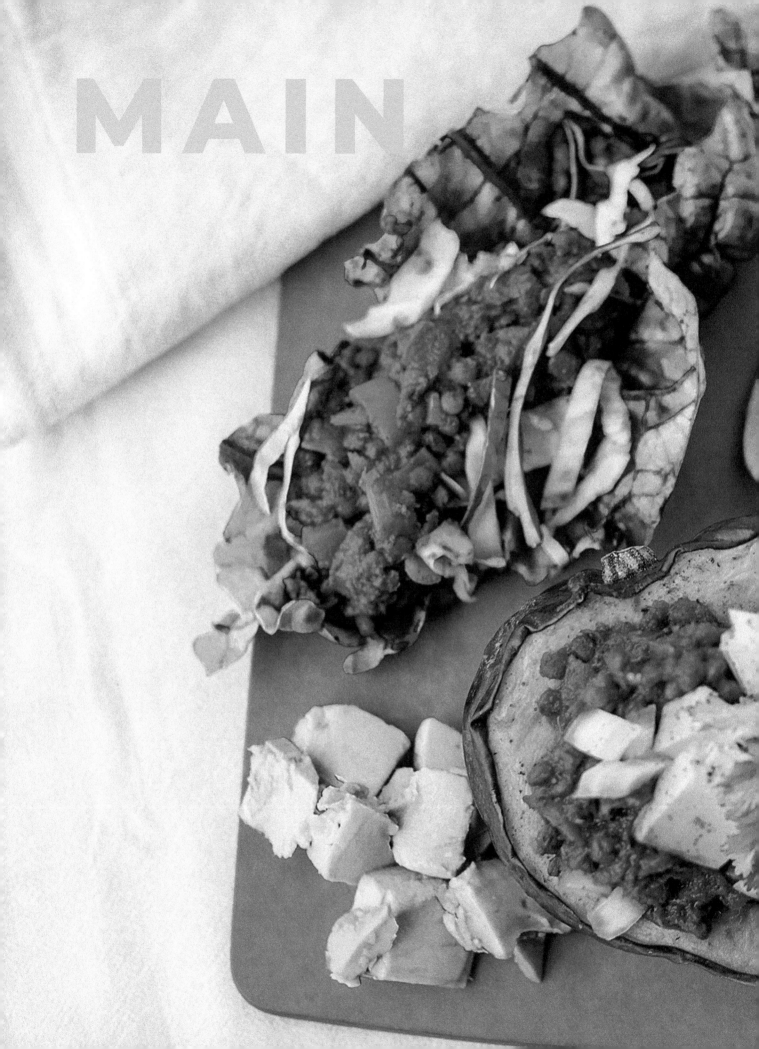

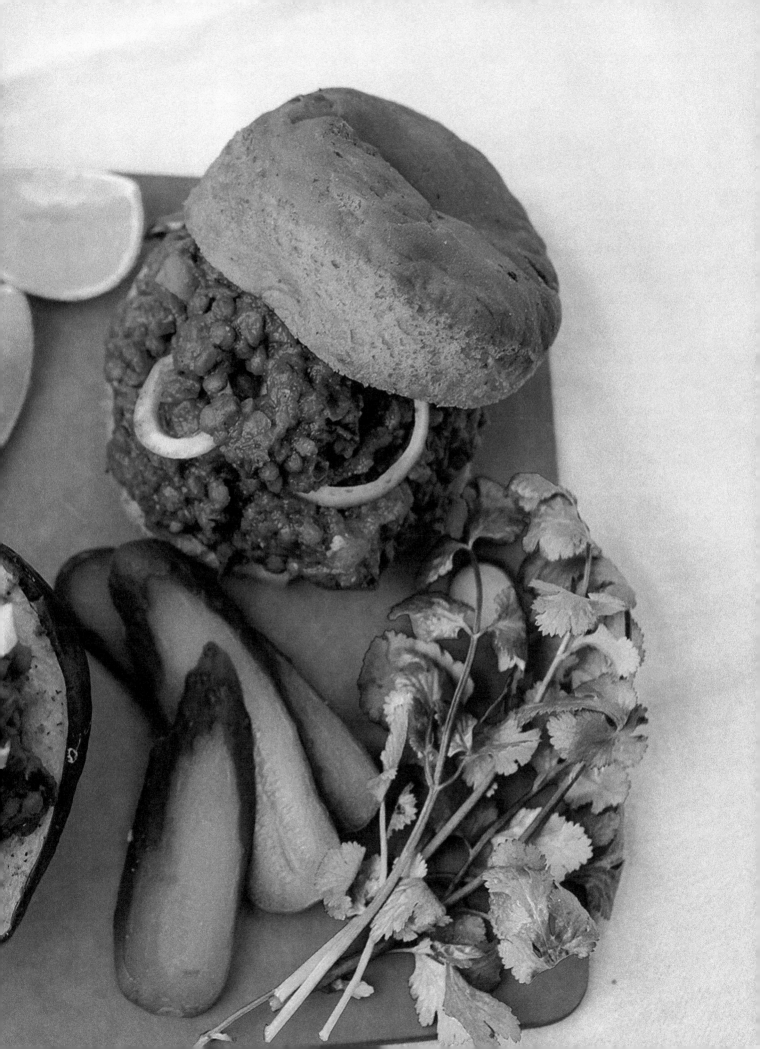

MAIN

Pulled Pork 2 Ways

INGREDIENTS

- Can of jackfruit
- Garlic powder
- Parsley
- Salt
- Thyme
- Smoked paprika
- Black pepper
- Cumin
- Onion powder
- Cayenne pepper
- Maple syrup
- Stone ground or dijon mustard
- Olive oil

DIRECTIONS

Open and drain the jack fruit and throw it in a large sauté pan with a drizzle of olive oil. Lightly sprinkle it with salt, black pepper, onion powder, thyme, cayenne pepper. Heavily sprinkle it with garlic powder, parsley, smoked paprika, and cumin. Add about 1 TBSP of maple syrup. Remember, real, dark maple syrup not the shitty corn syrup kind. Add about 1 teaspoon-ish of mustard and mix well. Cook until warmed through and the seasonings start to smell nice. Taste and adjust seasonings.

Nic loaded his "pulled pork" onto a nice toasted vegan bun and topped it with vegan mayo and spinach with a side of our vegetable medley.

Calie loaded her "pulled pork" onto a bed of greens topped with the vegetable medley and drizzled with buffalo sauce.

OPTIONAL ADD INS

1. Baked beans on the side or on top
2. Diced yellow onion
3. Thin strips of sauteed multi-colored bell peppers
4. A heaping scoop of vegan mayo based coleslaw for a true southern style pulled pork plate

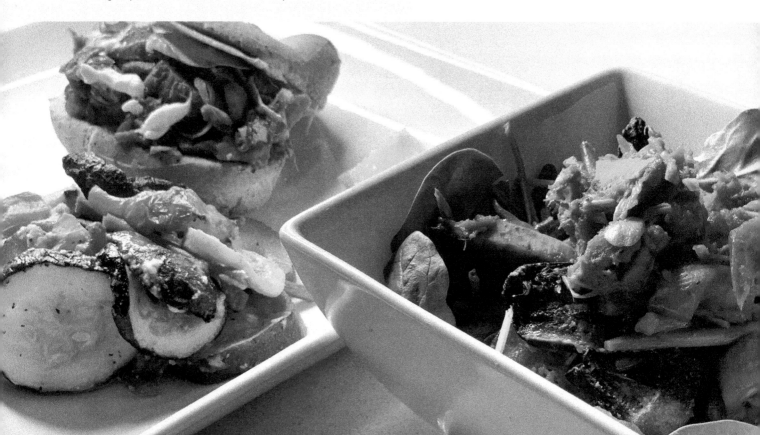

Ratings

lie - "So creamy and just e right amount of sweet from the squash."

Nic – "really light and filling."

 8

 8

Pairings

e - Lemon garlic broccolini

Nic – As is

In a small saucepan, while noodles are cooking. Warm about ¼ cup of your garlic parmesan sauce.

Transfer noodles to a bowl, top with parmesan sauce and sprinkle with chopped walnuts.

OPTIONAL ADD INS

1. This is so easy to change up by swapping your veggies (asparagus, broccoli, green peas, green and yellow zucchini...there are so many options!)
2. Swap the walnuts for pine nuts or pecans
3. Top with our vegetable medley and extra vegan parmesan cheese

Butternut Squash Pasta

INGREDIENTS

- Butternut squash "noodles" (buying them premade in the fridge or freezer section of the grocery store is definitely easiest, but you can use a spiralizer, it's just honestly a pain in the ass for such a hard vegetable)
- Spinach
- Tomatoes
- Walnuts
- Olive oil
- Salt
- Black pepper
- Garlic parmesan sauce

DIRECTIONS

Drizzle olive oil into a sauté pan and add your butternut squash noodles. Sprinkle with salt and black pepper and cook for about 10 minutes until heated through and softened. Add a handful of spinach and 3-4 small grape tomatoes. Sauté until both are wilted.

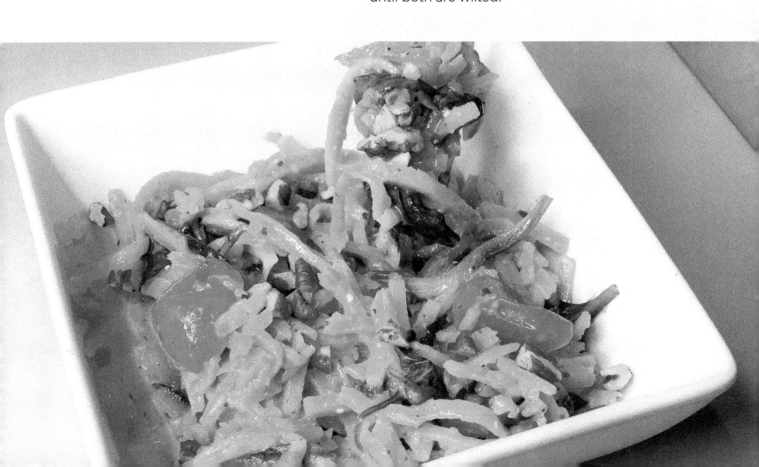

MAIN

Zucchini Lemon Garlic Pasta

INGREDIENTS

- Zucchini noodles (again, you can buy them pre-cut at the grocery store or spiralize them yourself. These are actually super easy because it's a softer vegetable.) Another simple option is to use a carrot peeler to create ribbon like zucchini strands for your "pasta"
- Asparagus
- Tomatoes
- Lemon
- Vegan butter (Earth Balance is our go to)
- Garlic
- Salt
- Black pepper

DIRECTIONS

In a large saute pan, add about 2 TBSP of butter, juice ½ a lemon, and 2 cloves of garlic finely chopped. Sauté for about 2-3 minutes on medium heat. Stirring so the garlic doesn't burn. Toss in your asparagus and cook for another few minutes before adding the zoodles and tomatoes. Sprinkle with salt and black pepper and cook until zoodles are heated and tomatoes are wilted.

OPTIONAL ADD INS

1. You can make this "heartier" by adding steamed lentils (seasoned with Italian seasoning mix or just garlic and onion)
2. Top with roasted chickpeas or cannellini beans
3. Crumble a clean, minimal ingredient plant-based veggie burger on top
4. Swap out the veggies to change it up. Roasted broccoli with nutritional yeast is a really flavorful and filling add in

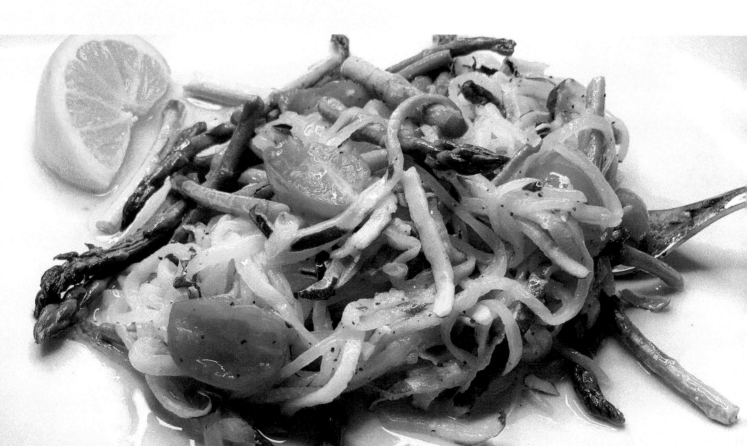

Ratings

alie - "So heavy for me... I eat ½"

 8

Nic - "Fuck yes, give me two"

 10

Pairings

Calie – "Tri-color fries"

Nic – "Yeah, Calie's Tri-color fries"

Portobello Steak Sandwich

INGREDIENTS

- Portobello mushroom
- Onion
- Orange bell pepper
- Vegan French baguette (use whatever bread you like and can find)
- Pineapple
- Sweet chili dipping sauce
- Olive oil
- Balsamic vinegar
- Salt
- Black pepper
- Garlic powder
- Vegan butter

Toss your bell pepper, pineapple and onion in olive oil with salt and pepper and grill or sauté.

Toast your bun with a little vegan butter. Top with mushrooms, bell peppers and onions. Optional: add the grilled pineapple or serve on the side.

Use our sweet chili dipping sauce or sauce of your choice for extra flavor because everything's better with sauces!

OPTIONAL ADD INS

1. Pickles
2. Coleslaw
3. Sauerkraut

DIRECTIONS

Thinly slice the portobello mushroom and marinate with olive oil, balsamic vinegar, and a sprinkle of the salt, pepper and garlic powder. Grill your mushrooms or put in the oven at 400 degrees for 30 minutes.

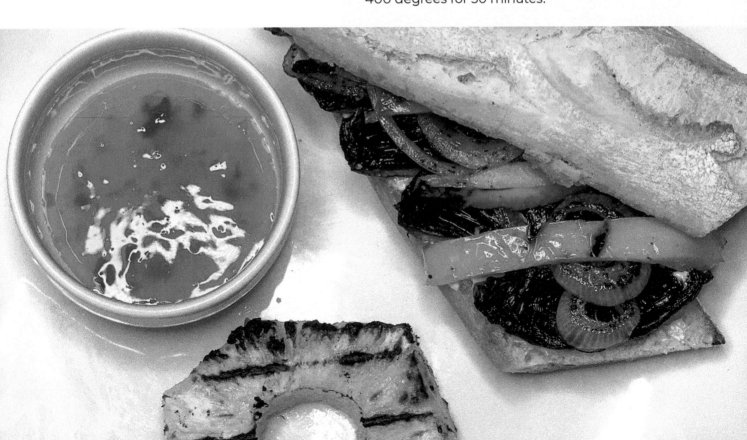

MAIN

Carrot Ginger Soup

INGREDIENTS

- About 1 lb of whole carrots
- 1 clove of garlic
- 2 TBSP of apple cider vinegar
- 1 cup of water or vegetable broth
- 1 TBSP of freshly grated ginger (it's worth the effort)
- 1 heaping TBSP of coconut butter (can substitute full fat coconut milk)
- Salt

DIRECTIONS

Combine the carrots, garlic, vinegar, and water or vegetable broth in a small sauce pan. Cover and bring to a boil, then lower the heat and simmer until your carrots are tender.

We let the carrots get a little charred on the bottom, which adds a really lovely flavor to the puree in the end. You don't have to.

Transfer the mixture to a blender or food processor and puree until smooth.

Return the puree to the saucepan and reheat, stirring in the ginger and coconut butter until well blended. Add salt to taste.

OPTIONAL ADD INS

1. Mix in roasted cauliflower and spinach
2. Pour it over zucchini noodles or glass noodles as a "sauce" with water chestnuts and snap peas

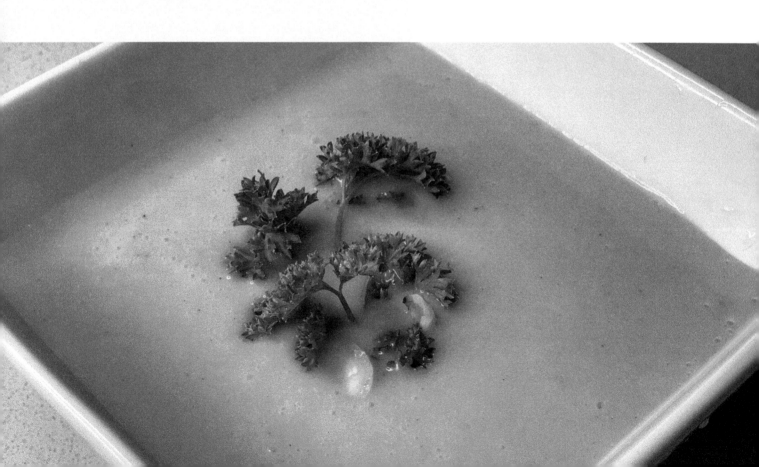

lie - "Mmmmmmmm"

10

Nic - "Not a tomato soup fan but this one was good"

6

MAIN

Fire Roasted Tomato Soup

INGREDIENTS

- 8-10 roma tomatoes
- 7 cloves of fresh garlic, peeled
- Olive oil
- Salt
- Black pepper
- ¼ of a yellow onion
- About 1/4 cup of vegetable broth
- ½ can of full fat coconut milk
- 3-4 fresh basil leaves

DIRECTIONS

Preheat oven to 425.

Slice roma tomatoes into quarters and drizzle with olive oil and sprinkle with salt and pepper. Place them on a baking sheet with garlic cloves and roast for about 30-40 minutes until skin is slightly browned and bubbling.

In a large saucepan add a drizzle of olive oil and onion slices and cook for about 5-7 minutes until slightly browned.

Add tomatoes, garlic, onion and vegetable broth to a blender or food processor and blend until completely pureed.

Pour tomato mix into a large saucepan.

Add coconut milk and basil to the blender and puree. Then pour basil coconut milk mixture into the large saucepan with your tomato puree. Heat until well mixed and taste test. Add salt or more basil as needed.

OPTIONAL ADD INS

1. Top with toasted cashews or pine nuts
2. Added roasted red peppers with your tomatoes
3. Mix in rice to make it heartier and more filling on it's own
4. Add cooked elbow macaroni and lentils

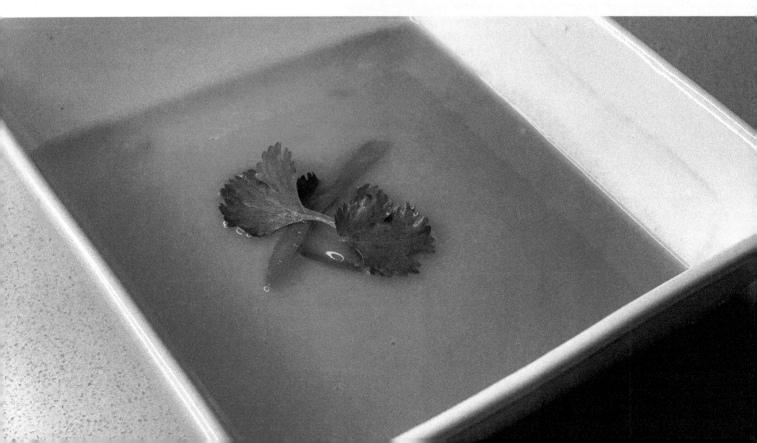

MAIN

Sweet Potato Quesadillas

INGREDIENTS

- Fajita veggie
- 1 can of drained and rinsed black beans
- Brown rice tortilla wrap
- Purple sweet potato mashed
- Orange sweet potato
- Spinach
- Smoky tempeh
- Vegan provolone and cheddar cheeses
- Vegan sour cream or vegan ranch
- Olive oil
- ½ TBSP chili powder
- 1 tsp paprika
- 2 tsp cumin
- ¼ tsp oregano
- ¼ tsp garlic powder
- ¼ tsp onion powder
- Salt
- Black pepper

DIRECTIONS

Preheat oven to 425. Slice your orange sweet potato into ¼ inch thick slices and drizzle with olive oil. Place on a baking sheet with a whole purple sweet potato and bake for 30 minutes. Flip the orange sweet potato slices after 15 minutes. Take the orange sweet potato slices out and cook the purple sweet potato for 10 more minutes.

While the purple sweet potato is finishishing, add olive oil to a saute pan and toss in your black beans, smoky tempeh, spinach. Sprinkle with the spices and saute for about 5 minutes until everything is warmed through.

Put provolone cheese on one wrap and cheddar on the second wrap. Place in your preheated oven for 5 minutes or until crisp.

Remove your purple sweet potato. Cut in half and spread the potato mash on one wrap. Top with orange sweet potato slices. Then add your fajita veggie mix and finally top with your tempeh, spinach and black bean mix. Add your second wrap to the top and cut in half.

Serve with vegan sour cream, vegan ranch or salsa.

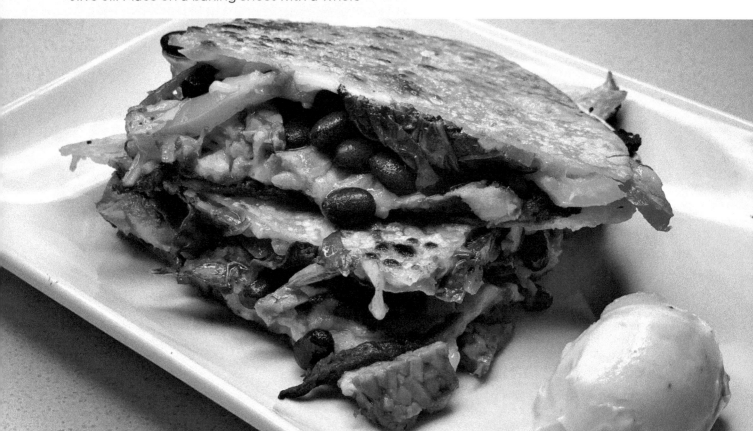

Ratings

Calie - "Solid"

 7

Nic – "really liked the seasoning on this one"

 8

Pairings

Calie - You could easily add some ground turkey or ground beef to one, two, or all of these to appease any non plant-based eaters.

Nic - I added ground beef

DIRECTIONS

Boil rice (just use the package directions). Cut Peppers in half and scoop out the seeds. Place on a baking tray and drizzle with oil and seasoning. Bake for 15 minutes at 415 degrees. While they're baking, cut the veggies into small pieces and saute with oil and seasonings for about 5 minutes. Add a few heaping TBSP of tomato sauce or salsa of your choice (we used an organic salsa). Mix in the rice and transfer mixture to the peppers. Place back in the oven for another 5 to 10 minutes. Add cheese to the top if you prefer or sprinkle with nutritional yeast for those B vitamins!

MAIN

Stuffed Italian Bell Peppers

INGREDIENTS

- Bell Peppers
- Rice
- Mushrooms
- Zucchini
- Tomato sauce (salsa, marinara, tomato paste)
- Onion
- Spinach
- Seasonings of your choice (We used Flavor God's Vegan Bacon Seasoning mix, Salt and Garlic)
- Olive Oil
- Optional: Vegan cheese or nutritional yeast

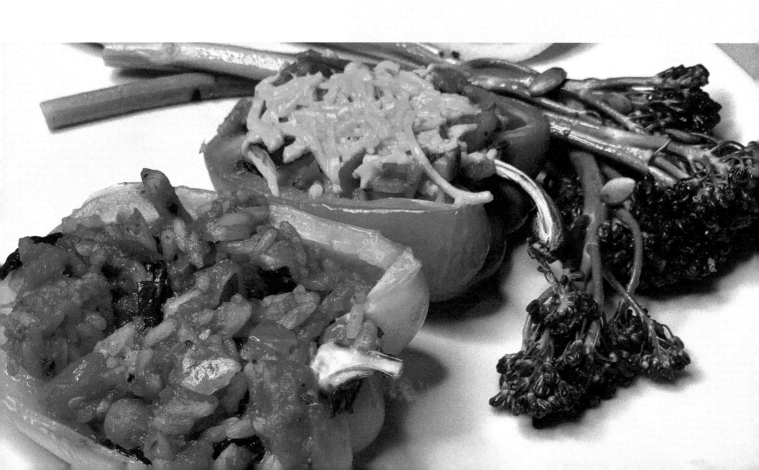

MAIN

Zucchini Taco Boats

INGREDIENTS

- 2 large zucchini
- About 1 cup of cooked lentils (red, green, any color works) OR Mushrooms and onion mince (just chop them up and cook in olive oil with salt and pepper)
- Olive oil
- Tomatoes
- Vegan cheese
- Cilantro
- ½ TBSP Chili powder
- 3 tsp Cumin
- 1 ½ tsp Paprika
- ½ tsp Garlic Powder
- ½ tsp Onion powder
- ½ tsp Oregano
- Salt
- Black pepper to taste
- Optional: Red pepper flakes

DIRECTIONS

Preheat oven to 400 degrees. Slice your zucchini down the center and use a spoon to gently scoop the seeds out of the center making room for the taco stuffing. Place on a baking sheet and drizzle with olive oil and sprinkle with salt and pepper.

Bake for 15 minutes so it's soft in the center but still solid enough to pick up and eat when stuffed.

While your zucchini halves are baking. In a large saute pan, drizzle a little olive oil and place your lentils or mushroom mince and season with taco seasoning blend. Stir and continue cooking until warmed through. About 5-8 minutes.

Remove your zucchini from the oven. Stuff each half with your taco mix. Top with cheese and place back in the oven for 5 minutes to melt cheese.

Remove from the oven and top with any taco toppings. We used tomatoes and cilantro.

OPTIONAL ADD INS

1. You can use our fajita veggie mix to stuff the zucchini boats for a more veggie heavy dish.
2. A crumbled plant-based veggie burger works as a stuffing in a pinch
3. Non-plant based eaters can you shredded chicken or you could use vegan "ground beef"
4. Roasted chickpeas cooked in the taco seasoning and mashed are also a great stuffing here

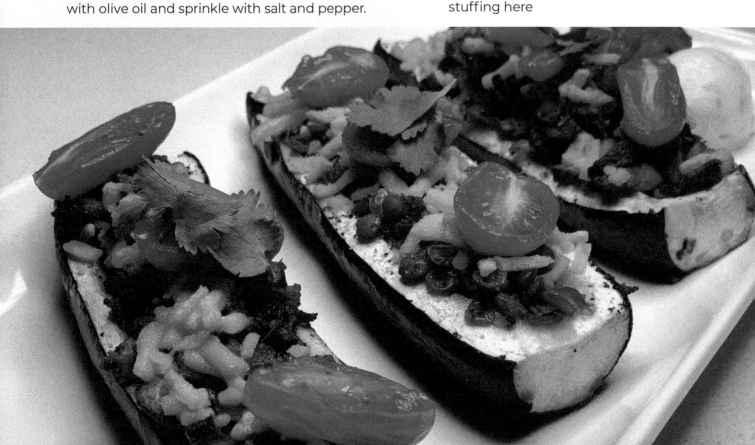

Hasselback Potato with Creamy Mushrooms

While the potato is cooking. Cut your mushrooms in half and toss them in a saute pan with about a few TBSP of our cashew cream sauce. If you don't want to make that recipe or don't have it on hand you can use a drizzle of olive oil plus 1 TBSP of vegan mayonnaise or coconut cream and season with black pepper, salt and 1 TBSP of nutritional yeast.

Remove the potato from the oven and pour creamy mushrooms over top or serve on the side.

Obviously, Calie adds hot sauce.

OPTIONAL ADD INS

1. Try using vegan mayo or coconut cream in place of the vegan butter on your potato.
2. Change up the seasoning to change up the flavor. Curry seasoning mix is a delicious option.
3. Add finely chopped herbs to your potato while cooking. Chives, rosemary, thyme are all great options.

INGREDIENTS

- Yukon Gold or Russet Potato
- Vegan butter
- Olive oil
- Salt
- Mushrooms (handful per potato)
- Cashew Cream Sauce

DIRECTIONS

Preheat oven to 420 degrees. Wash and dry your potato and cut ¼ inch slits in the top of the potato, but don't cut all the way through. Just about ½ way down. Drizzle with olive oil then press vegan butter between each slit.. Sprinkle with salt and pepper and make sure to open the slits so some seasonings get in between.

Place in the oven on a baking sheet and bake for about 30 minutes.

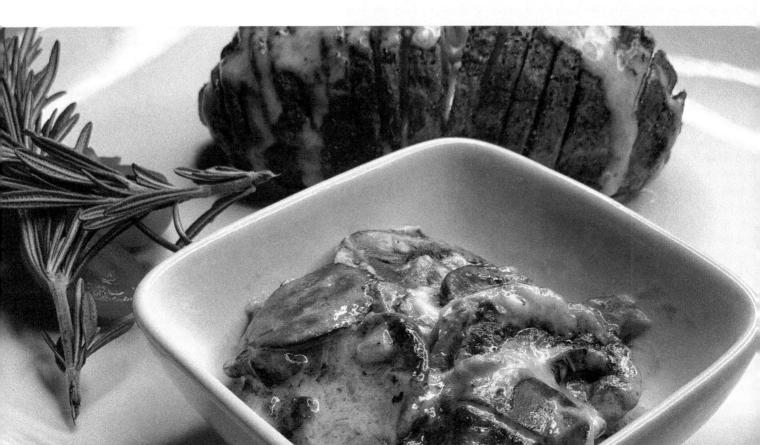

MAIN

Creamy Seaweed Pasta

INGREDIENTS

- Blue Evolution Superfood Seaweed Pasta (glass noodles or gluten-free soba noodles are great in this too)
- Asparagus, chopped
- Mushrooms, thinly sliced
- Toasted cashews (5-8)
- Fresh tomatoes or warmed up canned fire roasted tomatoes (that's we used for more flavor)
- Garlic parmesan sauce
- Olive oil
- Trader Joe's Everything But the Bagel Seasoning Blend (or similar mix of your own)

DIRECTIONS

Cook your pasta to package directions.

While the pasta is cooking, sauté your asparagus and mushrooms in a little olive oil and season lightly with seasoning mix. Cook for about 6-8 minutes to maintaining some crispness in your asparagus.

In a small saucepan, warm up desired amount of the garlic parmesan sauce. You can add the tomatoes right to it for convenience. Simmer for 5-8 minutes.

Ratings

Calie - I actually like this better with the tomato sauce from the eggplant lasagna. A little too filling for me otherwise.

 7

Nic – "Creamy goodne in a bowl."

 8

Drain your pasta and place it on your plate. Top wit sautéed veggies, sauce with tomatoes.

Toss your cashews in the sauté pan and toast for a fe min shaking the pan frequently to keep them from burning. Topps on top of your pasta and your done!

So many health benefits, in a super filling, comforting dish.

Optional: Layer all of these ingredients in a casserole dish adding a layer of spinach and bake for 20 minut Sprinkle wakame seaweed on top with the cashews and now you have a creamy, seaweed casserole you can serve to a large group with a nice side salad.

OPTIONAL ADD INS:

1. So easy to change up the veggies for variety. Broccoli and a few chopped shishito peppers are also delicious in this dish.
2. If you want it to be lighter swap the garlic parmesan sauce for the tomato sauce in the eggplant lasagna from Calie's Favorites.
3. Swap the seasoning blend for an Italian Mix or th Bragg's Sea Kelp Delight seasoning blend from Nic's Fish and Chips recipe

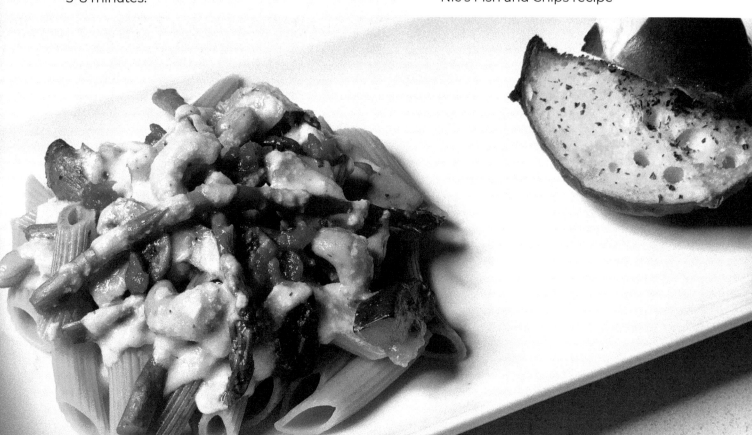

ie - "It's hard to beat my
ndma's meatball recipe,
but I do love these!"

Nic – "Love the flavor.
More sauce the better"

7   8

MAIN

Lentil Meatballs/Meatloaf

Pairings

alie - Meatballs with the
utternut squash pasta.
Meatloaf with the
Hasselback potato

Nic – Completely agree with
Calie on this one

INGREDIENTS

- 2 cups of precooked green lentils (or canned lentils)
- About a TBSP of olive oil
- 1 small yellow onion, diced
- 2 cloves of garlic, minced
- ½ cup of gluten-free rolled oats
- ½ cup of almond flour
- 3 TBSP of tomato paste
- 1 TBSP of Bragg's liquid aminos
- 1 TBSP apple cider vinegar
- 1 heaping TBSP of Italian seasoning mix

  OR

- Tsp each of oregano, basil and parsley
- ½ tsp each garlic powder and red pepper flakes
- Salt and black pepper to taste (you can taste it raw because it's not meat)

mond flour, lentils, cooked onions and garlic, tomato
aste, Bragg's, apple cider vinegar, and seasonings.
ulse a few more times to combine. Don't over process
it will be total mush and impossible to work with.

you haven't taste tested, this is your last chance. Add
easonings if necessary.

or meatballs, use a TBSP to scoop up your mixture and
ll it into balls. Arrange them on your baking sheet and
rush with a little olive oil

or meatloaf, press into loaf pan or muffin tin and we like
pour some of our smoky ketchup on top.

DIRECTIONS

In a sauté pan, drizzle about a tsp of olive oil, and sauté your onion and garlic for about 3 minutes. Then remove from the heat.

Preheat your oven to 400 degrees. Prepare a baking sheet with parchment paper if making meatballs or a muffin tin or loaf pan with a little coconut oil if making meatloaf or mini-meatloafs.

In a food processor or blender, add your oats and pulse a few times to make more of an oat flour. Add your

EATBALLS

ake for about 25 minutes. If you like your meatballs really
rispy on the outside you can bake for about 20 minutes
en toss them in your air fryer for 5 minutes at 350.

EATLOAF

ake for about 30 minutes.

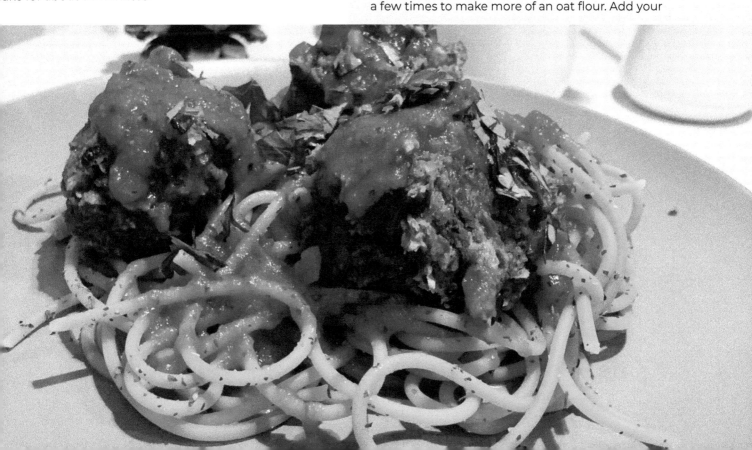

MAIN

Garlic "Butter" Mushrooms and Kale

INGREDIENTS

- 8 baby portobello mushrooms
- 2 TBSP vegan butter
- 2 TBSP full fat coconut milk with the cream
- Kale - about two stalks destemmed, and leaves chopped
- 2 cloves of garlic thinly sliced
- Salt
- Black pepper
- Parsley

DIRECTIONS

In a large sauté pan, add your butter, garlic, coconut milk and sauté for about 2 minutes to let the garlic flavor infuse the butter. Add your mushrooms and season with salt, pepper and sauté about 8-10 minutes until mushrooms are cooked through. Toss in your kale and cook until kale is slightly wilted...about 2 more minutes. Remove from pan and sprinkle with chopped parsley. For how easy this recipe is, it's insanely delicious!

OPTIONAL ADD INS

1. You can easily add more veggies to this dish and just double the sauce recipe. Carrots, broccoli or snap peas would be a great addition to make it even more filling.
2. If you want it to be cheesier you can add a TBSP of nutritional yeast or vegan parmesan cheese.
3. But honestly, why mess with perfection!

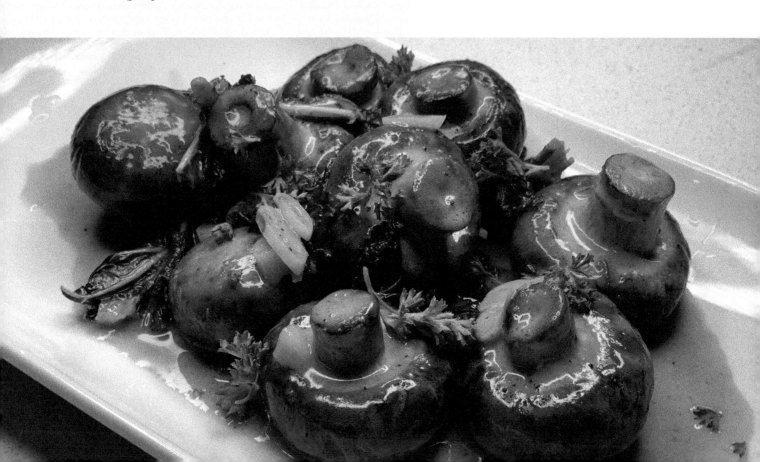

Ratings

MAIN

Chinese Stir Fry

INGREDIENTS

- Lotus Purple Rice (or any rice of your choice - Calie always uses cauliflower rice)
- Cup of Tofu
- Cup of Broccoli
- 1 Yellow Pepper
- Handful of cherry tomatoes
- ¼ cup Sweet and Sour Sauce
- Olive Oil
- Optional: Sesame oil
- Salt
- Pepper

DIRECTIONS

Boil your rice following the package directions. We feel like a broken record repeating that, but just in case you're wondering...unless you're using cauliflower rice. Then see below.

While your rice is boiling, cut your veggies and tofu. It really helps if you drain your tofu. Place it on a plate or a flat surface on a dish towel. Put another plate on top of it and gently press down or set something heavy on it for 10 minutes while you're chopping veggies and setting the rest of the recipe up. Drain the water from the plate or remove it from the towel and then chop.

ur recipe will come out much better without all
e excess water tofu holds.

ace a little olive oil (optional add in is a little sesame
) and toss in your veggies and tofu. Sprinkle with
asonings and saute for 12-15 minutes until the
ggies soften and turn a little brown. If you're using
uliflower rice, just throw it in the pan with the rest
your veggies and tofu.

dd sweet and sour sauce and saute for a further
to 3 minutes.

PTIONAL ADD INS

Swap the veggies if you don't like the ones we chose. We promise not to be offended.

Add some more spices to enhance or change the flavor. Obviously Calie would say red pepper flakes, but ginger & garlic are also great additions to this dish. Don't forget red and green chilies. They're so good for you!

You could bread your tofu with a little bit of honey and crushed pecans or panko bread crumbs to change up the feel of the dish.

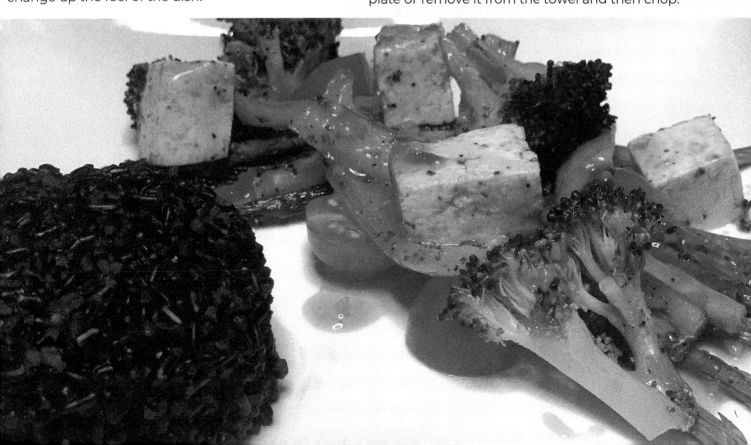

MAIN

Spring Rolls

INGREDIENTS

- Nasoya brand gluten free egg roll wraps (fridge section in most grocery stores)
- Broccoli/cabbage/carrot slaw mix (bought it pre-bagged)
- Bean sprouts
- Garlic
- Bragg's liquid aminos
- Olive oil
- Salt
- Black pepper

DIRECTIONS

In a sauté pan, drizzle about a tsp of olive oil, add a small handful of slaw mix per egg roll and a few thin slices of fresh garlic per roll. Sprinkle with Bragg's liquid aminos (or gluten-free soy sauce of your choice) and salt and pepper. Taste test for seasoning.

Warm through then remove from heat.

Lay your wraps out and place a heaping spoonful of your stuffing mix in the bottom corner. Roll once long ways. Fold the ends into the center to seal it then roll long ways until completely wrapped. Use a little water to make the end stick.

We "fried" them two ways. If you're going for the traditional, less healthy option. Pour about ¼ cup of olive oil in a small frying pan and heat over medium heat. Place your spring rolls in and cook on each side for about 2 minutes until golden brown. Remove at pat dry with a paper towel or kitchen towel to remove the excess oil.

The healthier option is to place your rolls in an air fryer. "Fry" them at 350 for about 10 minutes flipping halfway through.

Nic dipped his in a sweet and sour vegan chilli sauce and Calie dipped her in a mix of ½ dijon mustard and ½ honey.

Ratings

Calie – for the unhealthy fried version and a 9 for the healthier option. Can't go wrong!

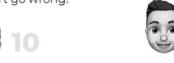

10

Nic – "Dip these bad boy the sauce multiple tim

10

Pairings

Calie - Vegetable medley or the broccolini for sure

Nic – Vegetable medle

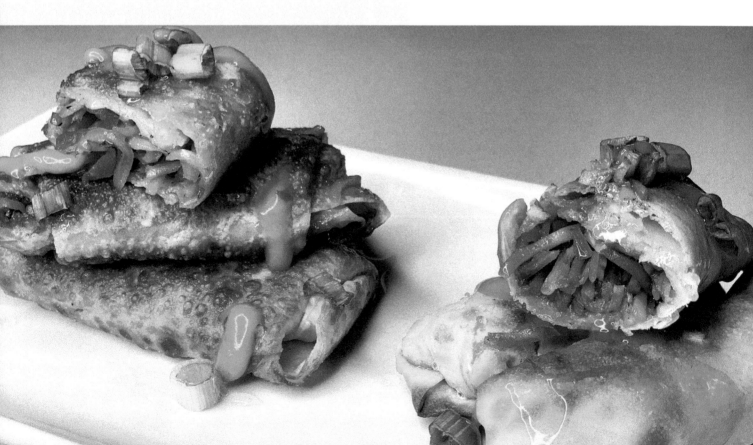

Ratings

Calie - "Better than Chinese take-out"

 9

Nic - "Filling and doesn't leave you feeling bloated"

 8

Pairings

Calie - Sweet chili edamame

Nic - Tofu Fries/nuggets

black pepper. Optional: add red pepper flakes. Cook stirring frequently for about 8-10 minutes until completely cooked through. Taste test and add more coconut aminos and seasoning if needed.

Remove from pan and top with chopped green onions to serve. Optional: add sesame seeds.

OPTIONAL ADD INS

1. If you aren't 100% plant-based you can add an egg or chicken
2. The leftovers are great in an egg roll wrap and fried or "air fryed" for a egg roll
3. Bamboo sprouts are a nice addition

MAIN

Cauliflower Fried Rice

INGREDIENTS

- 1 bag of frozen cauliflower rice
- 1 bag of frozen mixed veggies (green beans, carrots, lima beans, green peas)
- Olive oil
- Sesame oil
- Coconut aminos
- 2 cloves of garlic, finely chopped
- Salt
- Black pepper
- Green onions
- Optional: red pepper flakes and sesame seeds

DIRECTIONS

In a large sauté pan, add a drizzle of olive oil and toss in finely chopped garlic. Sauté for about 1 minute. Add cauliflower and veggies. Sprinkle generously with coconut aminos, a little sesame oil and a little salt (coconut aminos are salty), and

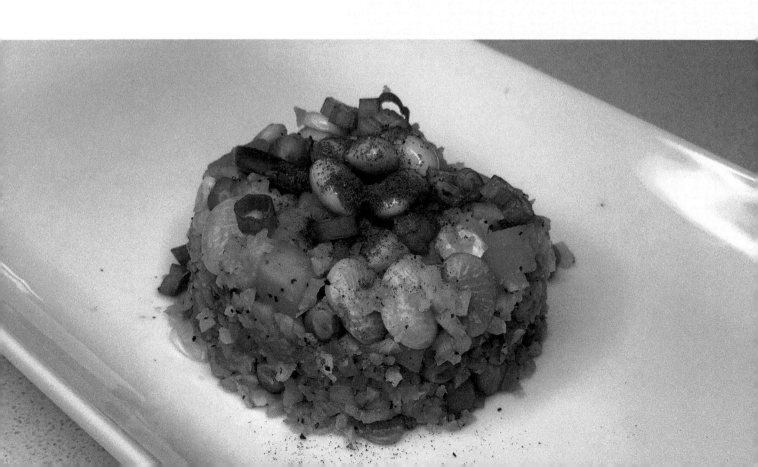

MAIN

Lentil Sloppy Joe's

INGREDIENTS

- 2 cups of cooked lentils or canned lentils
- Olive oil
- 1 small yellow onion, diced
- 2 cloves of garlic, finely chopped
- 1 small red pepper, diced
- Salt
- Black pepper
- 1 15 oz can of fire roasted tomatoes
- 1 TBSP tomato paste
- 1 TBSP of pure grade dark maple syrup
- 1 TBSP of vegan Worcestershire sauce (it's still good if you have to leave this out)
- 2 tsp of chili powder
- 1 tsp cumin
- ½ tsp of smoked paprika

Ratings

Calie - "Sloppy Joe's was never my favorite but this has great flavor."

 8

Nic – "Not my cup of tea this"

4

Pairings

Calie - Tricolor fries

Nic - Bloomin onion

DIRECTIONS

Cook your lentils according to package directions if you're making them from dry.

In a large sauté pan, add olive oil and toss in your garlic and onion. Cook for about 3 minutes stirring frequently. Add your bell peppers, and cook another 3-5 minutes. Toss in your lentils and remaining ingredients. Cook stirring frequently over medium high heat until you get a gentle boil. Reduce the heat to medium and let it cook for about 10 minutes stirring occasionally.

Serve on a vegan bun, open face vegan slice of bread, stuff it in a cooked acorn squash or even in your taco boats in place of "taco seasoned filling".

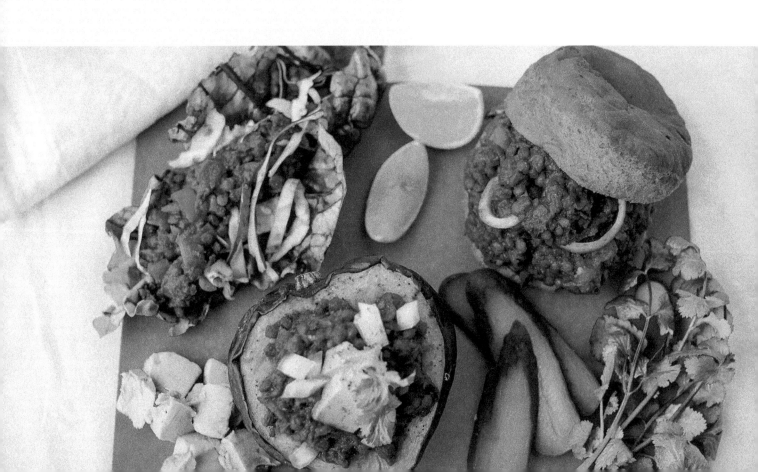

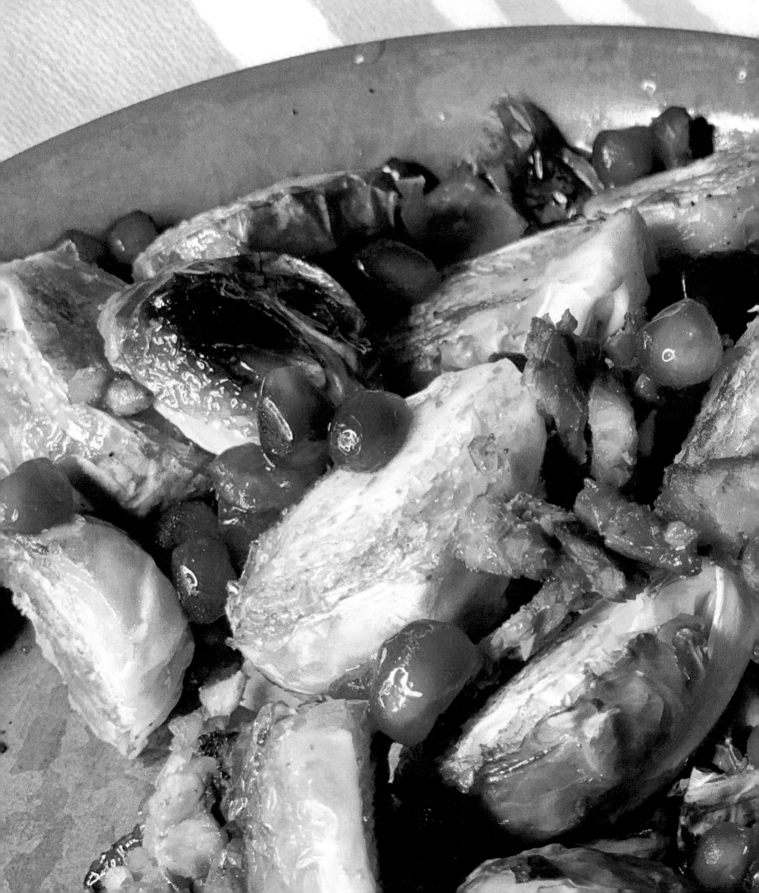

SIDES

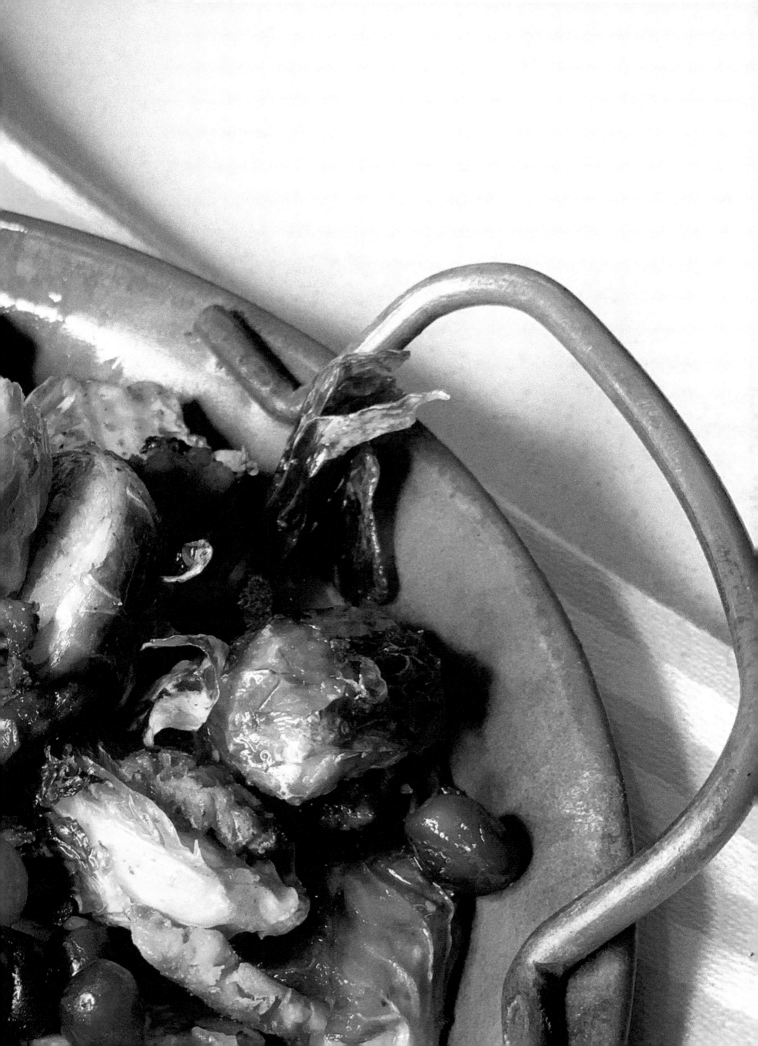

SIDES

Smokey Sweet Brussel Sprouts

INGREDIENTS

- 1 bag of brussel sprouts, halved
- Olive oil
- Maple syrup
- Salt
- Black pepper
- 2 strips Smoky tempeh bacon, crumbled
- Pomegranate seeds
- Optional: Buffalo sauce

DIRECTIONS

Preheat the oven to 425 degrees.

Cut the ends off the brussels, peel the outside leaves off and slice in half long ways.

Plae the brussels in a large baking dish and drizzle with olive oil and maple syrup. Sprinkle with salt and pepper and mix with hands until well coated.

Bake in the oven for 35-40 minutes on the top rack stirring once about half way through.

While the brussels are baking. Warm up two strips of smoky tempeh, crumbled.

Remove your brussels from the oven, sprinkle with smoky tempeh and top with pomegranate seeds.

Optional: drizzle a little buffalo sauce or hot sauce to kick it up a notch.

OPTIONAL ADD INS

1. Toast some almonds or pine nuts and toss them on top for a little extra flavor, crunch and protein/healthy fats.
2. You could use regular bacon if you aren't exclusively plant-based.
3. If pomegranate seeds aren't in season, try dried cranberries or raisins.

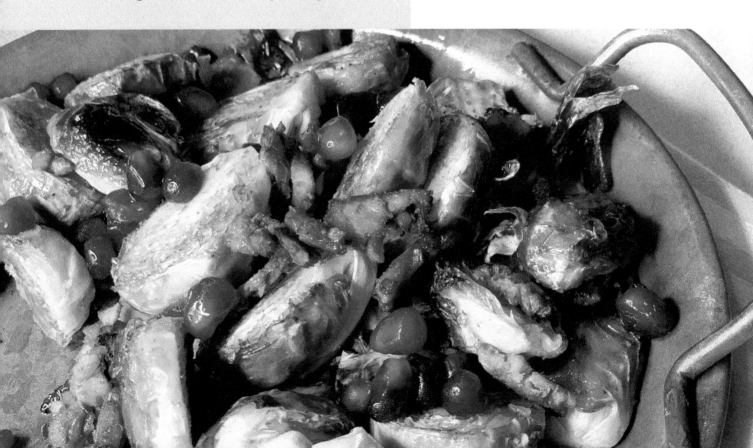

Ratings

Calie - I literally make ese 3 times a week. I'm sessed! Best thing Nic very introduced me to. He gets all the credit!

 10

Nic – You're welcome Calie

 10

Pairings

Calie - Lentil meatloaf

Nic – Literally any meal

Remove your carrots from the boiling water and place them in a large baking dish. Drizzle with olive oil and sprinkle heavily with your seasoning mix. Stir them up to coat all sides and bake for 35-45 minutes depending on how done you like them. We usually go 45 minutes to get them soft on the inside with a nice crisp on the outside and to let the natural sugars in the carrots caralize a little.

OPTIONAL ADD INS

1. We never doctor these up but we do love to dip them in hummus or other sauces.
2. You could add sauteed greens like spinach or kale.
3. Mix other root veggies in with them using the same directions like parsnips or beets.

SIDES

Roasted Carrots

INGREDIENTS

- 2 full size carrots per person (we like to use the tri-color bag because the colors have different flavors)
- Olive oil
- Seasoning mix of your choice. We usually go for either curry powder (both of our favorite) or a Cajun seasoning mix. Flavor God's Cajun seasoning blend is really good and so is their Everything Spicy Blend.

DIRECTIONS

Choose your carrot colors. White are the most bitter or earthy, purple are the sweetest and you guys know what an orange carrot tastes like (we hope) lol. Cut the ends off and chop them in half.

Place them in a large pot, completely covered with water, and bring to a boil. Turn the heat down and low boil for about 20 minutes.

While the carrots are boiling, preheat the oven to 420 degrees.

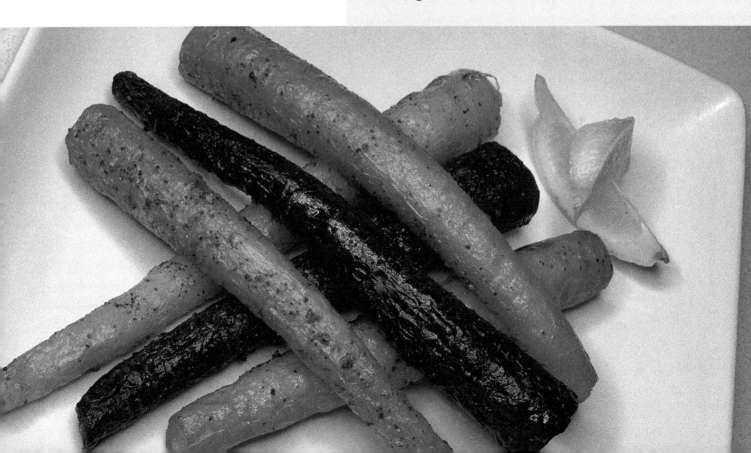

SIDES

Tofu Fries/Nuggets

INGREDIENTS

- Extra Firm Tofu
- Breadcrumbs
- Corn Starch
- Seasonings of your choice (We used Bacon Seasoning, Salt and Garlic)
- Chives
- Olive Oil

Ratings

Calie - I don't like tofu as much as Nic, but this might be my favorite way to prepare it.

 8

Nic - "Burst in your mou

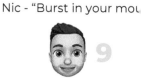 9

Pairings

Calie - Peanut sauce

Nic – Smokey Ketchu

DIRECTIONS

Don't forget to start by pressing the excess water out of your tofu. It's really important for the recipe or you'll get soggy fries.

Cut Tofu into cubes (or the length of a fry if you wanted them longer). Mix together the cornstarch and seasonings on a plate. Spread the breadcrumbs out on a separate plate and season them heavily as well. Roll the tofu cubes in the corn starch seasoning mix, then drizzle with oil, then roll in the breadcrumbs. Drizzle a pan with olive oil and turn the heat up to medium/high, sear for around 45 seconds per side.

If you have an air fryer, you can just toss the in there at 350 for about 15 minutes turning once half way through.

Drizzle with lemon and sprinkle of chives. Pair with your favorite dipping sauce.

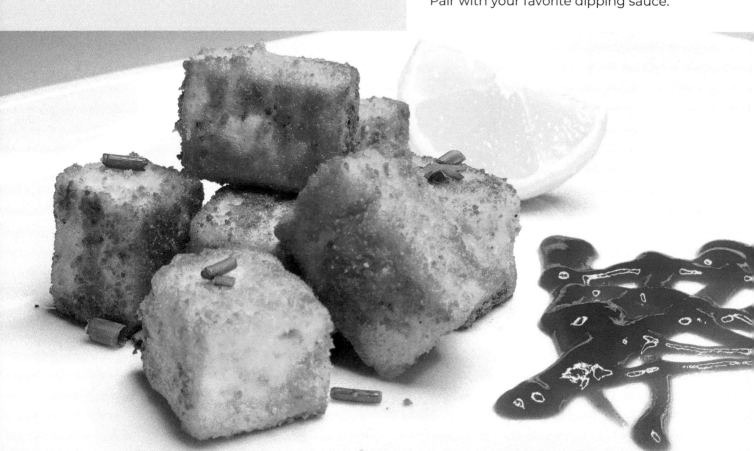

ie - we use these in a lot
other recipes, but they're
great on their own.

Nic – a go-to side for sure.

10

9

Pairings

lie - Roasted chickpeas

Nic – Balsamic Mushrooms

SIDES

Fajita Vegetables

INGREDIENTS

- Red bell pepper
- Yellow bell pepper
- Orange bell pepper
- ½ yellow onion
- ½ red onion
- Olive oil
- 1 TBSP chili powder
- 3 tsp of cumin
- 1 ½ tsp of paprika
- ¼ tsp each of oregano, garlic powder, onion powder
- Salt
- Black pepper
- cilantro

DIRECTIONS

Preheat your oven to 425 degrees.

Very thinly slice all of your veggies. Almost julienne. Google it and you'll see what we mean :)

Place them in a large glass baking dish and drizzle with olive oil. Sprinkle all of your seasonings on top then use your hands to really mix it well. Make sure all the veggies are coated.

Bake it in the oven for about 30 minutes. Mix once or twice so they cook evenly.

Top with some chopped cilantro and you're done.

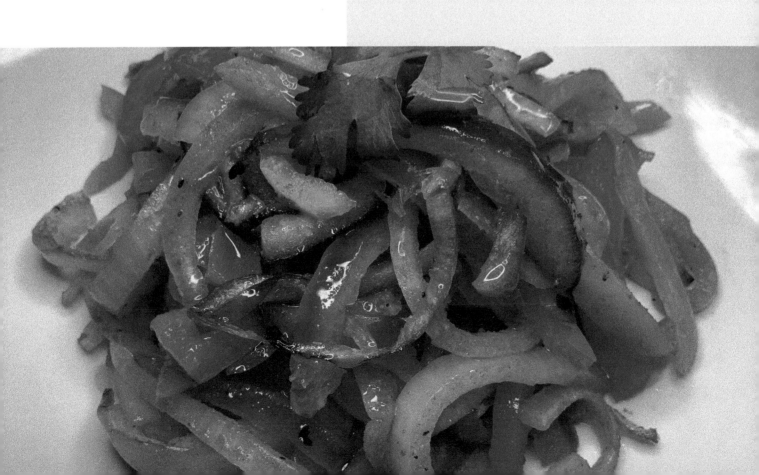

SIDES

Lemon Garlic Broccolini

INGREDIENTS

- 1-2 bunches of broccolini (it's different than broccoli, although if that's all you can find you can use broccoli)
- Olive oil (or vegan butter for richer flavor)
- ½ a lemon
- 1 clove of garlic, peeled and thinly sliced
- Salt
- Black Pepper
- Optional: red pepper flakes (just Calie...ok)

DIRECTIONS

Drizzle a large saute pan with olive oil or about a TBSP of vegan butter. Toss in your garlic and cook for about 2- 3 minutes stirring continuously.

Add your broccolini and squeeze the lemon juice on it. Sprinkle with seasonings and cook about 3 minutes per side or up to 5 if you like it with a little brown.

Ratings

Calie - it doesn't even make it to my plate. I eat it straight out of the pan.

 10

Nic – love the lemon flavor on these

 9

Pairings

Calie - Portobello Steak Sandwich

Nic – Supergreen Burg

We think it's best crispier and bright green. Overcooking it makes it limp, soggy and hard to eat.

OPTIONAL ADD INS

1. Sesame seeds, pine nuts, pumpkin seeds... you get the idea.
2. Olive slices (not the black ones though...try kalamata)
3. Fire roasted bell peppers (you can get them in a jar and just slice them up and toss them in.)

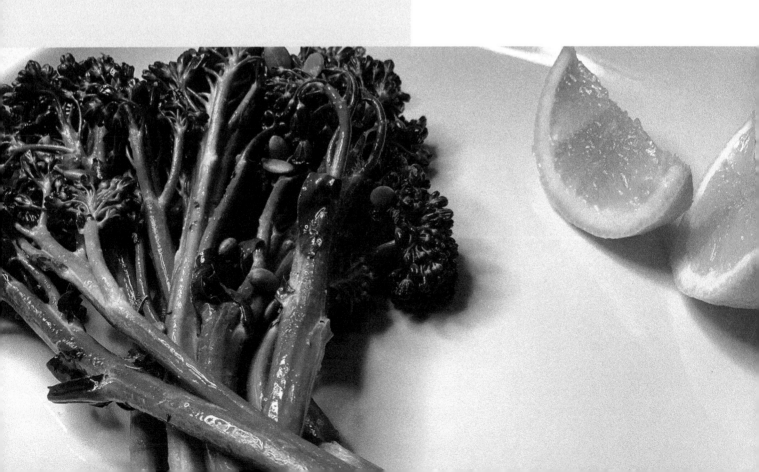

Ratings

alie - best snack, I pack
ese in my kids lunches,
out they prefer turkey
acon from Applegate

10

Nic - Crunchy and
filling

8

Pairings

ie - Super Green Burger

Nic – Chinese Stir Fry

DIRECTIONS

Preheat the oven to 425. Cover a baking sheet in parchment paper.

Layout out two strips of tempeh bacon next to each other. Put 4-5 green beans at the end of the strip, tuck the bacon up around it and roll.

Lay each bacon green bean cluster and lay it on your baking sheet.

Bake for 40 minutes flipping ½ way through.

SIDES

"Bacon" Wrapped Green Beans

INGREDIENTS

- Smoky Tempeh Bacon (or you can make eggplant bacon...but you'll have to google a recipe because it didn't make the cut for book 1 lol)
- Green Beans

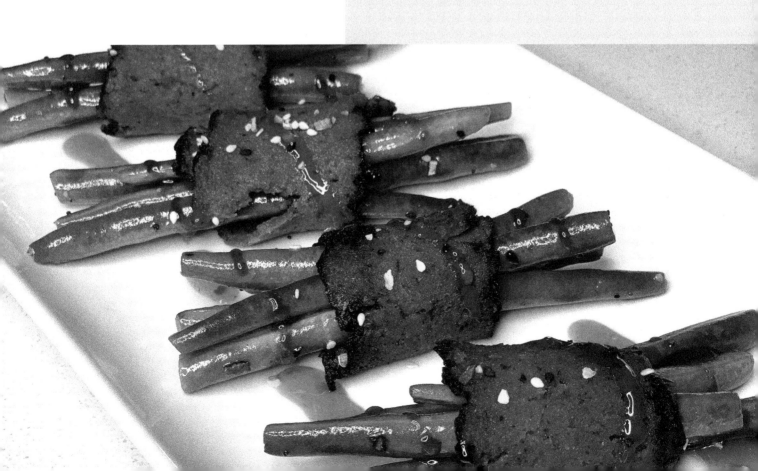

SIDES

Kale Chips

INGREDIENTS

- 1 bunch of kale (someone asked us what this means in one of our groups...kale is sold in bunches when it's not pre-chopped and bagged. That's what you're looking for. Chopped kale shrivels up into nothing.)
- ½ a lemon
- Olive oil
- Salt
- Black pepper

Ratings

Calie - the boys and I literally fight over these

 10

Nic – I eat these four tir a week minimum

 10

Pairings

Calie - Leftover Hot Dogs

Nic – Literally anythin

DIRECTIONS

Preheat your oven to 325 degrees. Line a baking sheet with parchment paper.

Wash your kale and thoroughly dry it. Chop the extra stem at the bottom off. Place all of your kale in a bowl and drizzle lightly...lightly people or it won't turn into a chip! Sprinkle with a little salt and pepper.

Bake for about 30 minutes flipping halfway through.

Squeeze the lemon juice on top and munch away.

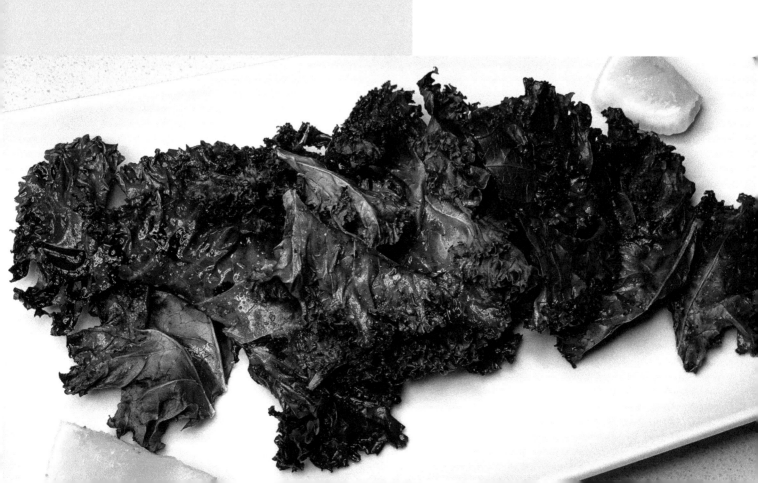

Ratings

Calie - restaurant quality...love serving this for parties or making as a Saturday afternoon movie snack

9

Nic - "I ate them all"

10

Pairings

Calie - Radicchio Salad   Nic – Creamy Seaweed Pasta

DIRECTIONS

Preheat oven to 400.

In a small bowl combine your olive oil, balsamic vinegar and seasonings. Add your mushrooms and toss to completely coat.

Transfer to a glass baking dish and roast in the oven for about 25 minutes.

OPTIONAL ADD INS

1. You can use a variety of flavored balsamic vinegars
2. Change up the spices adding thyme or rosemary

SIDES

Balsamic Mushrooms

INGREDIENTS

- 8-10 baby portobello mushrooms, halved
- About 2 TBSP olive oil
- About 2 TBSP high quality balsamic vinegar (it should be more syrup like than vinegar like in consistency)
- Salt
- Black pepper
- Garlic powder
- Fresh parsley

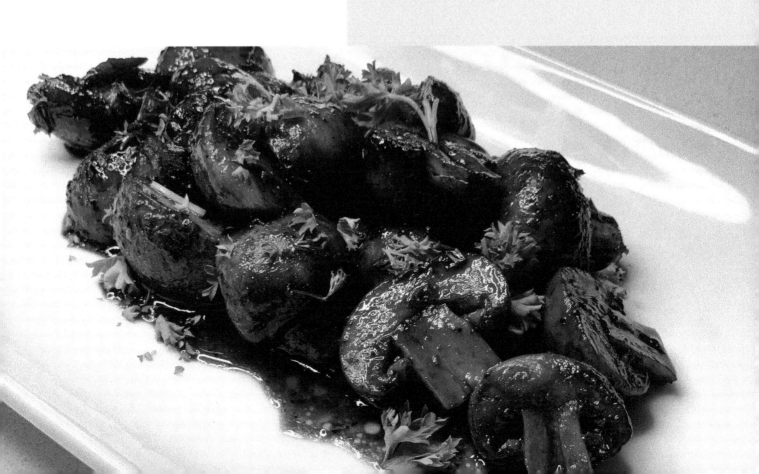

SIDES

Chickpea Chicken Salad

INGREDIENTS

- 1 can of organic chickpeas, rinsed and drained
- 4-5 fresh sage leaves (rosemary is good too)
- Salt
- 2 stalks of celery, thinly sliced
- About 1/4 cup of olive oil
- About ¼ cup of Apple Cider Vinegar
- 1 tablespoon vegan Dijon mustard
- Paprika
- Black pepper
- Sliced almonds or chopped walnuts
- Handful of chopped green apple

DIRECTIONS

Add chickpeas, sage, and salt to your food processor. Pulse until crumbly. You can leave chunks for a more "chicken" salad like texture or pulse longer for a smoother consistency. Also, we are lazy cooks so we just mix it in a bowl and don't bother processing it all, but the texture is nicer if you do.

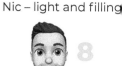
Scoop your chickpea mixture into a large glass bowl and add the remaining ingredients. Mix well. I think it's best chilled so I like to put it in the fridge for a few hours before serving. I recommend doubling the recipe because this salad is good on everything, including salad, and it goes quickly.

OPTIONAL ADD INS

1. If you want it to be creamier, substitute vegan mayo for the olive oil and acv
2. Swap the apple for grapes, cranberries, pears...whatever you have or feel like
3. How you eat it is where you have the most room for creativity. On crackers, with bell pepper scoops, on zucchini boats or cucumber slices, in a sandwich with cheese and toasted???? So many options.

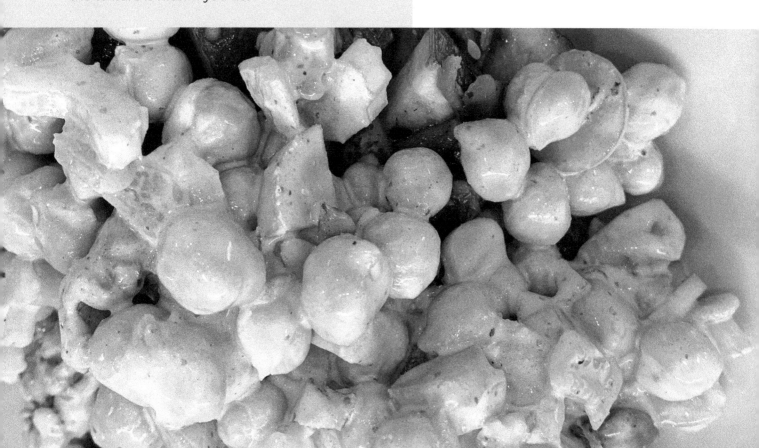

Ratings

Calie - perfect texture...
the sauce makes them!

 8

Nic - more seasoning
the better

 8

Pairings

Calie - Tacos

Nic – Supergreen Burger

DIRECTIONS

Cut avocado into about 8 wedges. Pour breadcrumbs onto a plate and season heavily with salt, pepper and paprika. You should be able to smell the seasonings.

Drizzle the avocado wedges with olive oil and make sure they're lightly coated on all sides.

Roll the wedges in the bread crumb mix and pat it tightly until it stick in a thick layer.

Transfer to your air fryer and cook at 400 for 8 minutes.

Drizzle with lemon juice and dip in salsa, ketchup or your favorite dipping sauce.

SIDES

Avocado Fries

INGREDIENTS

- Avocado sliced into wedges
- Gluten free breadcrumbs
- Salt
- Black pepper
- Paprika
- Olive oil
- Lemon

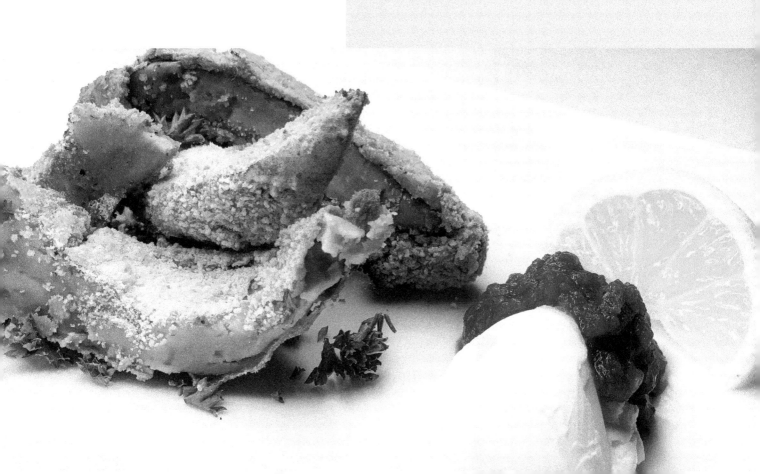

SIDES

Radicchio Salad

INGREDIENTS

- 1 small radicchio
- Primal Kitchen Honey Mustard Dressing
- Vegan mayo
- Stoneground Mustard
- Green peas (pre-cooked, steamed)
- Chili lime pistachios (or nut of your choice), deshelled and chopped
- Treeline Chipotle Serrano Pepper Soft Cheese
- Cilantro
- Cholula Sauce

DIRECTIONS

Quarter your radicchio.

Place it on a plate - inside facing up. Sprinkle your green peas on top.

Chop up your pistachios or nuts of your choice and sprinkle on top. Crumble some of your Treeline cheese on top.

In a small bowl, mix about 1-2 TBSPs of your honey mustard dressing. Add about 1 tsp of vegan mayo and 2 tsp of mustard and mix with a fork.

Drizzle the dressing on top and sprinkle your fresh cilantro on (or herb of your choice).

This is a really filling salad with SO much flavor.

OPTIONAL ADD INS

1. You can add roasted veggies to the top of this for a bigger meal and to really make it a solid main dish.
2. You could easily add tuna or chicken.
3. Edamame in place of green peas is also a good option.

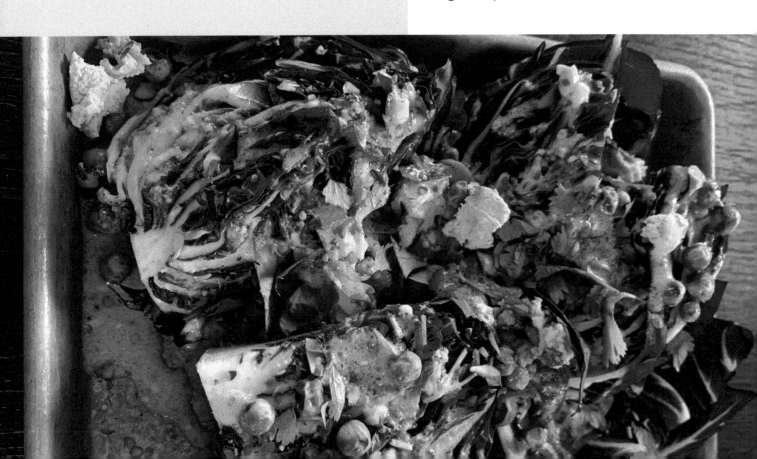

Ratings

Pairings

Calie - kabobs

Nic - Kabobs

SIDES

Greek Pasta Salad

INGREDIENTS

- 1 box 8 oz box of quinoa and rice elbow pasta (or any gluten free pasta)
- ½ a cucumber, chopped
- 8-10 cherry tomatoes, halved
- ½ a red bell pepper, diced
- 10 olives, halved
- ¼ red onion, diced
- ¼ cup of Miyakos sundried tomato and garlic soft cheese
- Parsley

DRESSING

- ¼ cup of red wine vinegar
- ¼ cup of olive oil
- Salt
- Black pepper
- Oregano

DIRECTIONS

Boil pasta to package directions, drain and rinse with cold water.

While it's boiling mix up your dressing in a small bowl. Seasoning to taste.

Transfer your pasta to a large serving bowl and toss all the ingredients in. Mix well and chill for at least an hour before serving.

OPTIONAL ADD INS

1. You can make this a creamy pasta salad by adding ¼ cup of vegan mayo or a ½ a mashed avocado.
2. Spice it up with a sprinkle of red pepper flakes
3. Make the onion flavor more mild by using a yellow onion.

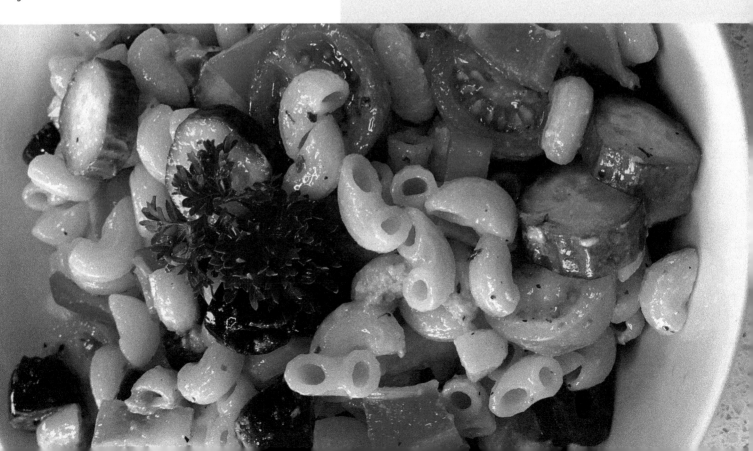

SIDES

Roasted Chickpeas

INGREDIENTS

- 1 can of chickpeas drained and rinsed (also called garbanzo beans)
- Olive oil
- Seasoning mix of your choice (per usual we tend to go with curry or cajun, but the taco seasoning blends from the fajita veggies is great on this too and you can't go wrong with salt and black pepper.)

Ratings

Calie - super diverse...I toss them in salads or just grab a handful as a snack

 9

Nic – easy and filling Better than popcorn

 9

Pairings

Calie - Savory popcorn

Nic – Sprinkle these o anything, especially sal

DIRECTIONS

In a large saute pan, drizzle a little olive oil. Pour your chickpeas in and sprinkle heavily with seasoning. Swirl them around in the pan to full coat in the flavors and turn the heat to medium/high.

Continue stirring while the chickpeas cook and keep cooking until a few start to pop like popcorn.

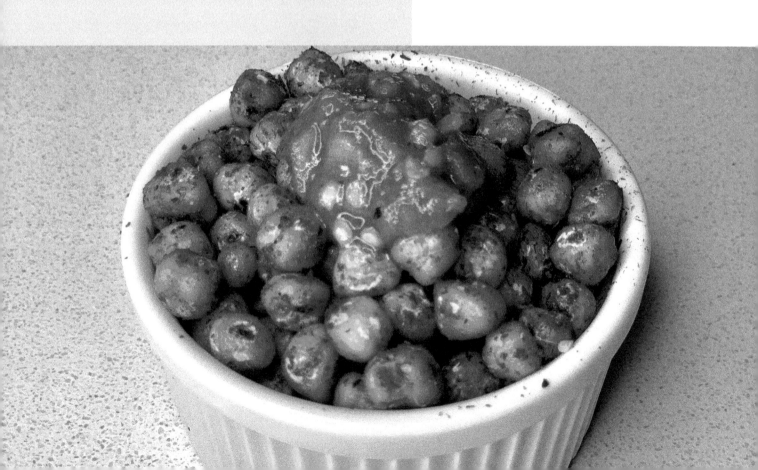

Ratings

Calie - mouth waters just thinking about it!

10

Nic – too good. Don't care that they are stuck in my teeth!

10

Pairings

Calie - Sweet Potato Quesadillas

Nic - Kabobs

DIRECTIONS

Preheat your grill.

In a large saucepan, boil water with a little dash of salt.

Remove corn from husks and add them to the boiling water. Boil for around 5 minutes.

Remove the corn from the pan and place it on a plate. Spray evenly with cooking oil, place on grill, turning them occasionally (every 1 to 2 minutes) with tongs. The corn will slightly brown.

Remove from the grill and brush all sides with mint yogurt sauce or just drizzle it over the top. Sprinkle each with 1 Tbsp. crumbled gouda cheese and squeeze 1 lime wedge over each ear. Sprinkle with a little paprika and chopped cilantro. Boom! Grill perfection.

SIDES

Street Corn

INGREDIENTS

- Corn
- Olive Oil Spray
- Salt
- Blak Pepper
- Paprika
- Gouda Cheese (Optional)
- Mint Yogurt Sauce
- Lemon or Lime juice
- Cilantro

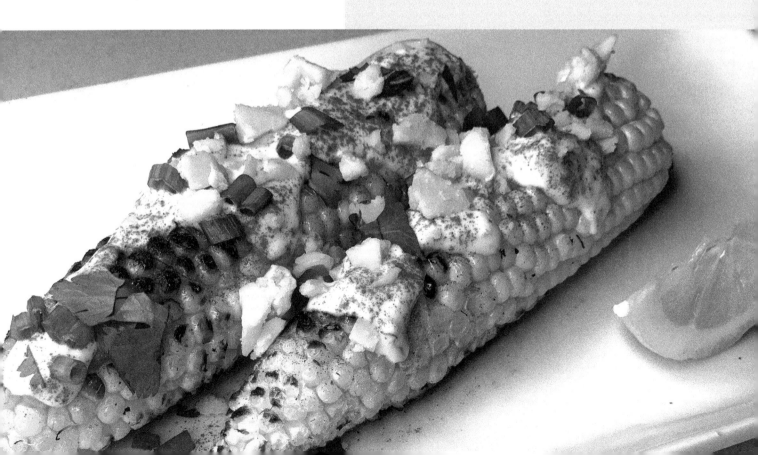

SIDES

Sweet Chili Edamame

INGREDIENTS

- Frozen organic edamame (however much you want based on if it's a side, a snack, a main...you decide)
- Marion's Coconut Sweet Chili Sauce (We like her sauce because it's vegan, gluten free, non-gmo and preservative free.

Ratings

Calie - sweet chili isn't my personal favorite. I like straight up coconut aminos or just salt on my edamame

 5

Nic – don't know why but Calie has somethi against sweet chilli.

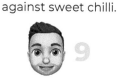 9

Pairings

Calie - Cauliflower rice bowl

Nic - Spring Rolls

DIRECTIONS

Place your edamame in a small sauce pan, cover with water and turn the heat up to medium/high.

Bring to a boil then turn off the heat and let them sit in the hot water for about 5 minutes.

Put them in a serving bowl and drizzle with sweet chili sauce.

Done! You don't always have to cook from scratch. Sometimes it's ok to have a little help from the good plant-based brands out there.

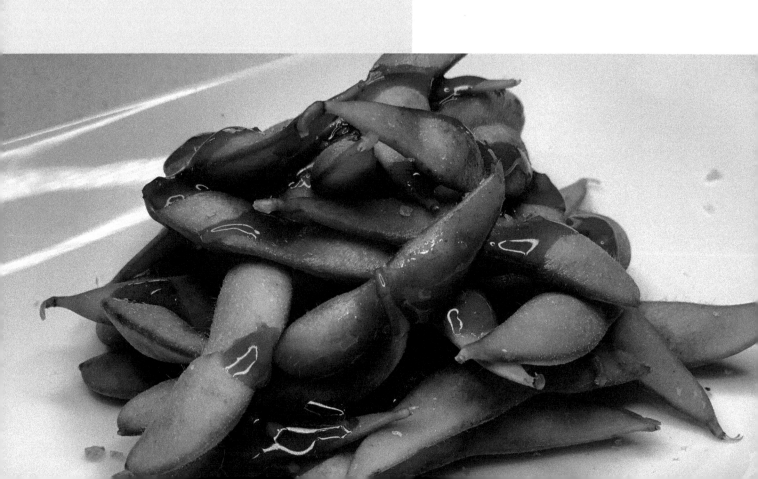

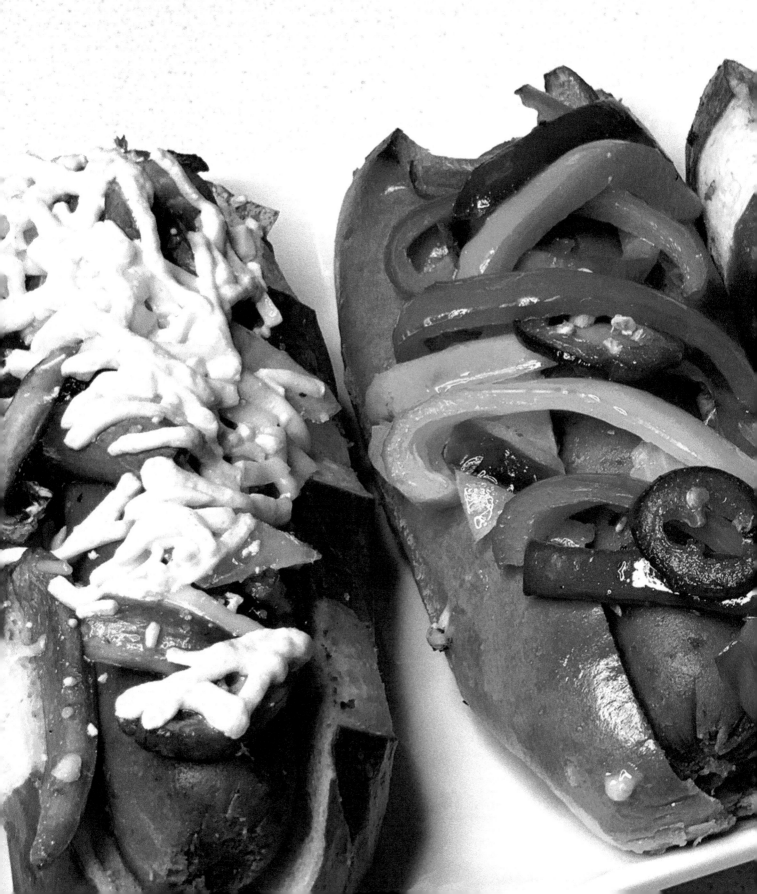

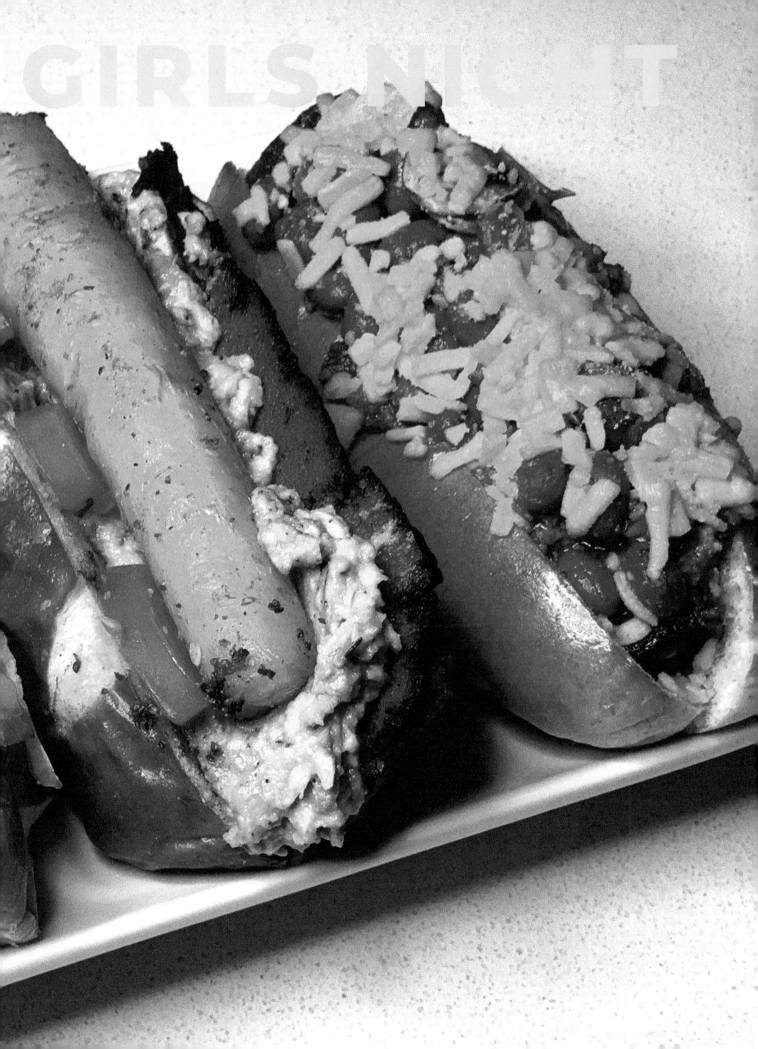

Crostini's

INGREDIENTS

- Baguette of choice
- Olive oil or vegan butter
- Shredded vegan cheese or soft cheese spread (Miyakos has great flavors)
- Tomato slices
- Fresh basil
- Pesto (we just use jarred, but it's easy to make your own if you want to try it and there are tons of recipes online...we only had so much room in this book)
- Salt
- Black pepper

DIRECTIONS

Preheat oven to 400 degrees.

Cut baguette into 1 inch thick slices and spread with olive oil or butter.

Add cheese & tomato slices and sprinkle with salt and pepper.

Ratings

Calie - damn it Nic! Quit making me love all the carbs. Just kidding... I eat carbs!

 10

Nic – dish these bad b[...] out at your next part[...]

 10

Pairings

Calie - Fire Roasted Tomato Soup

Nic – Any soup

Bake for about 10 minutes until golden and crispy.

Top with a dollop of pesto and a little fresh basil leaf. Sprinkle with salt and pepper.

OPTIONAL ADD INS

1. Change the sauce, change the flavor. Any of our sauces would be delicious for crostini. Just match the ingredients to match the flavor.
2. Nacho cheese sauce...add onions and bell peppers with cilantro and green chilies.
3. BBQ sauce...add jackfruit with taco seasonings, shredded vegan cheddar and jalapeno.

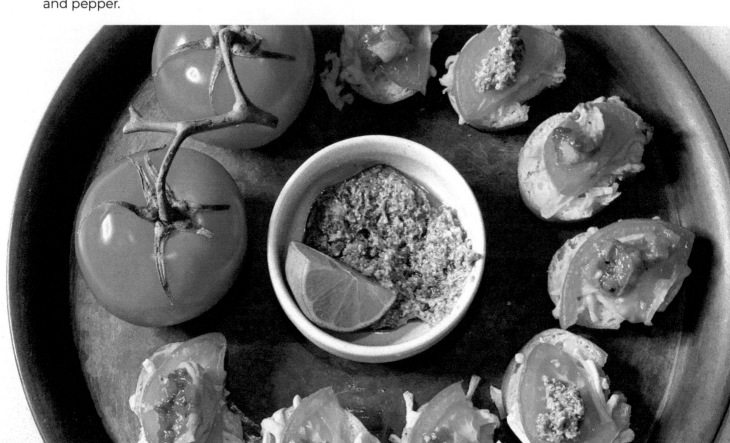

...lie - I love a platter. I do
...ese with leftovers all the
...me for the boys and we
...call it a picnic dinner.

Nic – 10, make any platter
that you want.
Easy and quick

 10

 10

Warm your tempeh bacon strips in a sauté pan.

Make your spinach and artichoke dip or use the lemon white bean hummus.

Prepare your crostini.

Lay all of your ingredients out on a large platter and you're ready to watch the game, sip wine with the girls or enjoy a movie night and hard kombucha.

OPTIONAL ADD INS

1. You can easily use all raw fruits and veggies and a store bought dip to make a much faster version of this platter, but we think the hot foods on here are worth the time....especially if you're having people over. Show them how great plant-based food tastes!

2. You can add some chips or the savory popcorn.

3. Olives are another great addition to these platters.

INGREDIENTS

- Grapes (we like ours frozen) or fruit of your choice
- Smoky tempeh bacon strips (heated in a sauté pan)
- Bell peppers
- Celery
- Green beans
- Mushrooms
- Spinach and artichoke dip
- Dark chocolate pieces
- Trail mix or raw nuts
- Crostini

DIRECTIONS

Put a little vegan mayo in a dish and sprinkle with salt and pepper. Roll the green beans and mushrooms in it. Then roll them in gluten free panko breadcrumbs. Toss them in your air fryer at 350 degrees for 15 minutes or in a 425 degree oven for about 20 minutes.

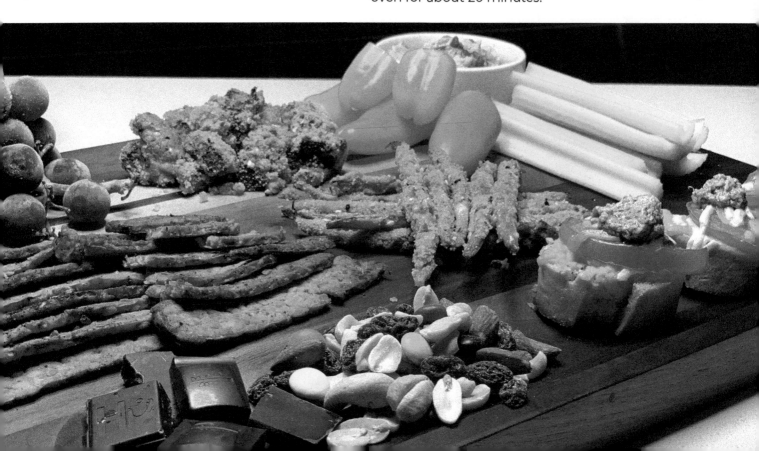

GAME DAY & GIRLS NIGHT

Hot Dogs 4 Ways From Leftovers

INGREDIENTS

- Hot Dog Buns of your choice (We used gluten free buns and pretzel buns and toasted them)
- Plant-based Sausage of choice
- Carrots
- Vegan Chilli
- Fajita veggie mix
- Garlic parmesan sauce
- Green bell peppers
- Smoky tempeh
- Vegan shredded cheese

DIRECTIONS

We wanted to show you guys some fun ways to use your leftovers that don't feel like eating leftovers! SO...we made 4 different hot dogs using leftovers from 4 different recipes in the book and some traditional hot dog toppings.

1. Garlic Parmesan Dogs - Cook your plant-based sausage according to package directions or use a roasted carrot. Place it in your bun. Top with garlic parmesan sauce, green peppers, and some shredded vegan cheese.
2. Fajita Dogs - Cook your plant-based sausage according to package directions. Place it in your bun. Top with fajita mix and buffalo sauce or sauce of your choice. Yum!
3. Carrot Dogs - Put your leftover roasted carrot in a hot dog bun, top with smoky tempeh bacon, mashed avocado with a little lemon juice, salt and pepper and tomatoes.
4. Chili Dogs - Plant based sausage cooked to package directions. Place it in a toasted hot dog bun and top with our vegan chili and shredded cheese.

You can use the carrots or plant-based sausage for any of these combos. This is just a group of ideas to help you get started. Add your favorite hot dog toppings to finish them off!

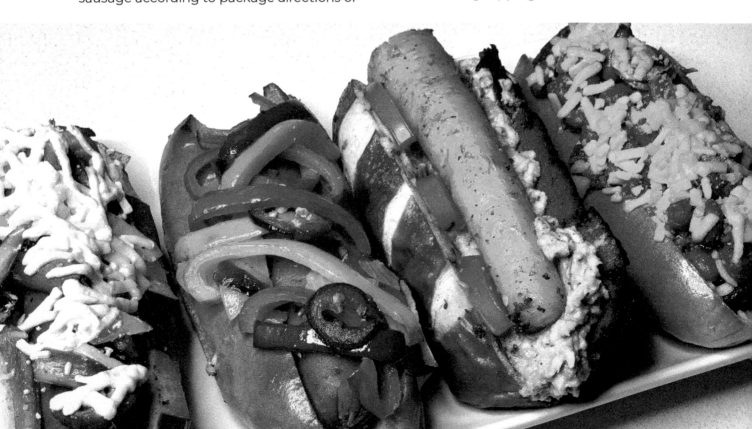

Loaded Sweet Potato

Ratings

Calie - a regular in my breakfast rotation but also ... to serve for a healthy but ...ng girls night main dish ...h a nice soup and wine.

 8

Nic – really hearty and I usually have this for lunch

 8

Pairings

...lie - Carrot ginger soup

Nic – As is

Once they're done cooking, toss a handful of kale into the pan with them and your onions and garlic. Drizzle with olive oil and sprinkle with salt, pepper, fennel and sage. Taste test it to make sure you seasoned it enough. Cook until kale is wilted and onions are translucent.

Remove your potato from the oven and slice down the center, but not all the way through. Add your chickpea and kale mixture to the center. Drizzle with a little nacho cheese sauce or top with a little vegan sour cream and chives.

OPTIONAL ADD INS

1. Add some smoky tempeh bacon or you could add an egg over easy if you aren't totally plant based or chopped turkey sausage.
2. Change the sauce and change up the flavor.
3. Swap the kale for our fajita veggies or just add those too!

INGREDIENTS

- Small sweet potato
- Roasted chickpeas
- Kale, chopped
- Onion, thinly sliced
- Garlic, thinly sliced
- Sesame Seeds
- Olive oil
- Salt
- Black pepper
- Fennel seeds
- Sage
- Chives
- Optional: Nacho cheese sauce

DIRECTIONS

Preheat your oven to 425 degrees. Pop your sweet potato in and let it cook for 25-35 minutes depending on how thick it is.

While your potato is baking. Make the roasted chickpeas with cajun style seasoning.

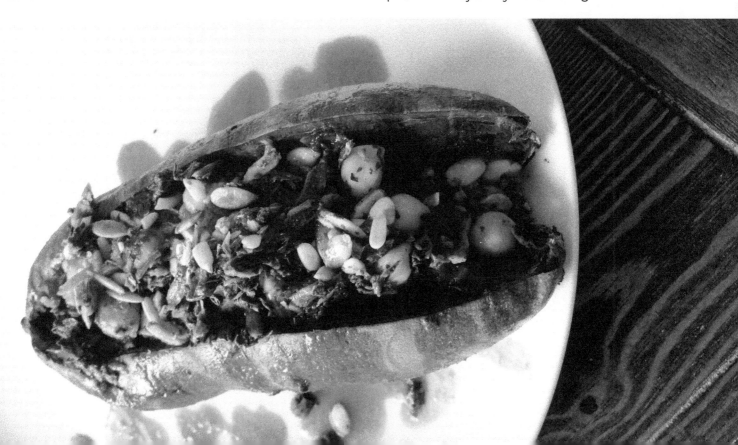

GAME DAY & GIRLS NIGHT

Mango Jalapeno Margarita

INGREDIENTS

- Jalapeno Infused Tequila (or just Tequila)
- Mango Gourmet Syrup
- Sparkling Lime Water
- Fresh Mango
- Fresh Jalapeno
- Lime Juice
- Margarita Salt
- Ice

DIRECTIONS

Add 1 shot of your tequila into a blender with a handful of ice. Add in a few chunks of fresh mango, one slice of jalepeno (more if you want it extra spicy), a shot of mango syrup and a teaspoon of lime juice. Blend.

Cover the top of a tall glass with margarita salt. Add a few ice cubes. Add your blended mix. Top it off with sparkling lime water (or just sparkling water). Garnish with a few jalapeno slices and mango for decoration and extra flavor.

Tip: wear gloves when working with the jalapenos otherwise you might end up with burning eyes and Calie laughing while you cry because you itched your eye. Anything you touch with jalapeno fingers (even after you wash your hands) just might end up burning. You've been warned!

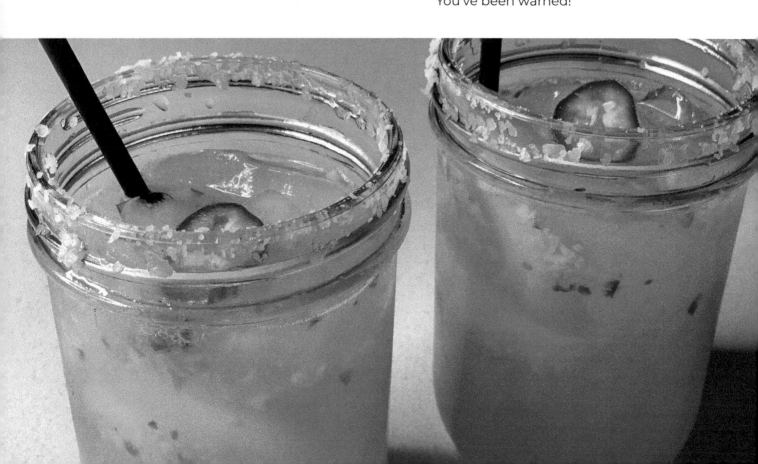

Super Green Burger

Ratings

ie - I love veggie patties
d this is by far one of the
I've had. I make lots and
ze them to use all month.

10

Nic – Amazing and filling.
The more items on this
the better.

9

Pairings

alie - Mango Jalapeno
Margarita

Nic – Tofu Fries

INGREDIENTS

- 1 cup of peas
- 1 cup of baby spinach
- ½ cup of broccoli florets blanched
- ½ cup of kale
- ½ cup chickpea flour
- ¼ cup of breadcrumbs
- 1 tsp cumin
- 1 tsp paprika
- Salt to taste
- Pepper to taste

DIRECTIONS

Put your green peas and broccoli in a blender and blitz them a few times. Transfer to a big bowl and add in the rest of the ingredients mixing with your hands....your clean hands...that you washed for 30 seconds. (We wrote this cookbook during COVID-19 so we couldn't not mention it.) Scoop out enough to shape into a burger size patty. How big and thick you like your burger is up to you. Calie uses about ¼ cup per patty and Nic uses double that. Put a drizzle of oil in a pan and cook until brown on both sides just like you would with a meat pattie.

Nic uses a bun because he is a bread-a-holic and Calie wraps hers in a collard green leaf because you can never get too many greens.

Top with your favorite burger toppings and condiments. Done!

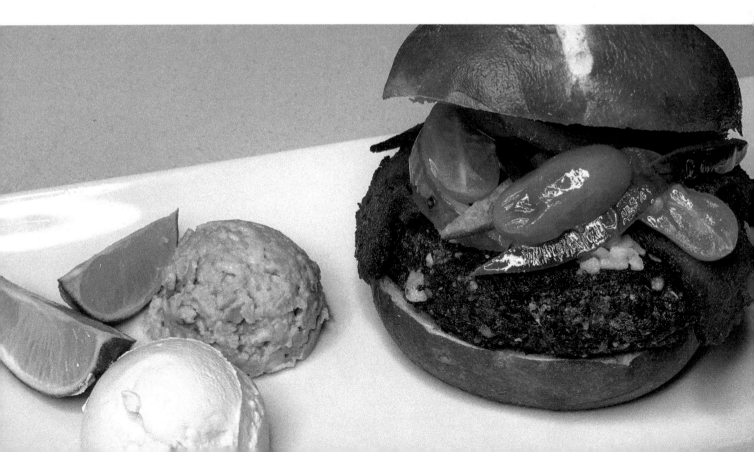

GAME DAY & GIRLS NIGHT

Buffalo Cauliflower Bites

INGREDIENTS

- Cauliflower (we like to get orange and purple and white...mix things up a little)
- Your favorite Buffalo Sauce (we go with Tessamae's or New Primal)

DIRECTIONS

Chop your cauliflower into large florets, rinse and pat dry.

Place it in a large bowl and drizzle it with buffalo sauce. Use your hands to mix it and make sure the florets are all well covered. Get it in the grooves!

Place in your air fryer at 375 degrees for about 15 minutes turning halfway through. We generally have to do a few batches to make sure it cooks evenly.

If you don't have an air fryer you can lay your florets on a baking sheet covered in parchment paper and bake at 425 for about 35-40 minutes until edges turn brown.

OPTIONAL ADD INS

1. You can also bread your florets by dipping them in the buffalo sauce and rolling them in a tiny bit of honey then in gluten-free breadcrumbs seasoned with a little chilli powder and paprika and maybe a dash of cayenne.
2. Turn these into loaded cauliflower nachos but putting our nacho cheese sauce on top with beans or shredded chicken if you eat that and adding traditional nacho toppings like onions, bell peppers and cilantro.
3. Use our BBQ sauce to make BBQ cauliflower bites the same way.

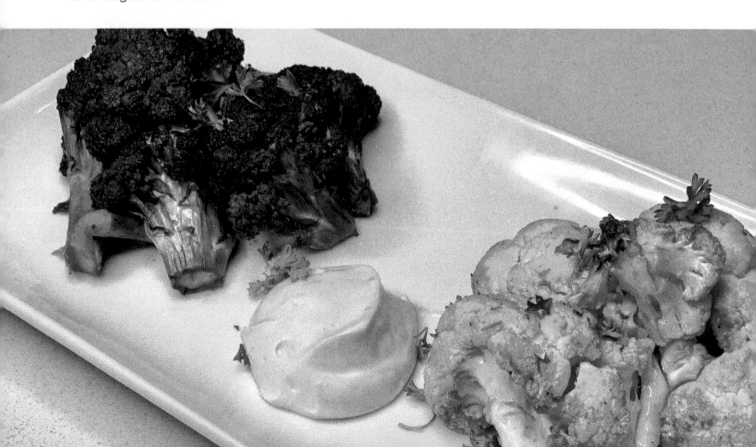

...lie - restaurant quality...
...e serving this for parties
...r making as a Saturday
...fternoon movie snack

9

Nic - "Bloody Brilliant"

10

GAME DAY & GIRLS NIGHT

Bloomin Onion

INGREDIENTS

- 1 large yellow onion
- Olive oil
- Curry seasoning blend (or seasoning blend of your choice)
- Gluten free breadcrumbs
- Foil
- ½ avocado
- 2 TBSP of vegan mayo
- Salt
- Black pepper
- Paprika
- Sweet chili curry sauce (store bought, or any hot sauce/buffalo sauce)

DIRECTIONS

Preheat oven to 425. Cut your onion into eights by cutting and X down the center without cutting all the way through. Then another X. Don't cut to the root or it will just fall apart. You want it to stay in tact so it opens up like a flower "blooming".

Drizzle it with olive oil and massage the oil into the crevices. Sprinkle your curry powder or seasoning of choice, opening each layer and making sure to rub into each layer.

Bake in the oven for an hour.

Remove from the oven and sprinkle with gluten free breadcrumbs. Press them all around the top and edges. Transfer to an air fryer and "air fry" the onion for 20 minutes at 380 degrees. This step is optional but gives it a nice crisp and is worth the effort in our opinion.

While it's "frying" mash ¼ an avocado and mix with about 2 TBSP of vegan mayo. Sprinkle in salt and black pepper to taste and top with a dash of paprika.

Remove your bloomin onion from the air fryer when it's done and drizzle it with sweet chili curry sauce. Pull apart and use as scoops for your avocado dip and thank us later!

OPTIONAL ADD INS

1. You can easily change this up with different seasoning blends. We love it with taco seasoning mix, simple salt and pepper or Trader Joe's Everything But the Bagel Seasoning mix.
2. Add shredded vegan cheddar cheese or sprinkle with parmesan cheese.

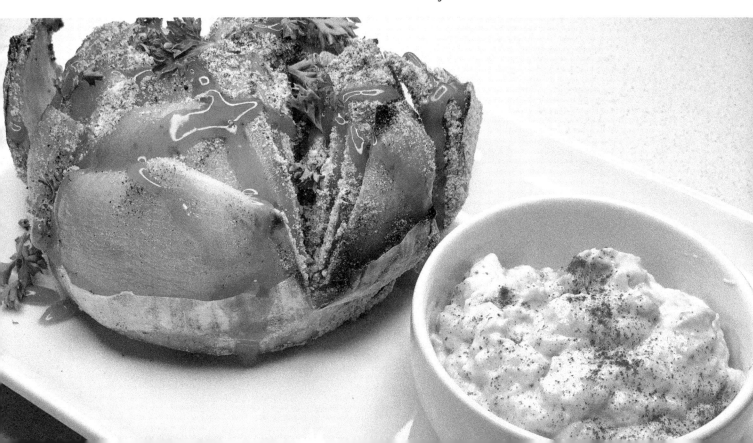

GAME DAY & GIRLS NIGHT

7 Layer Dip

INGREDIENTS

- 1 can of refried beans
- ¾ cup of salsa
- Spinach, chopped
- Red bell pepper, diced
- Vegan shredded cheddar cheese or our Nacho cheese sauce
- Vegan sour cream
- Olives
- Green onions, chopped
- Green chillies or diced jalapeno
- Cilantro, chopped

In a square glass baking dish or pie dish layer ingredients in order listed.

Serve with chips and by chips we mean anything crunch that can hold this amazing dip. Carrots, celery, bell pepper wedges, zucchini rounds or traditional tortilla chips or pita chips.

OPTIONAL ADD INS

1. Not sure how much more you could add to this, but if you eat meat you could add ground beef or chicken.
2. You could also optional add OUT any ingredients you don't like.
3. Really make the flavor pop by sprinkling the top with taco seasoning mix.

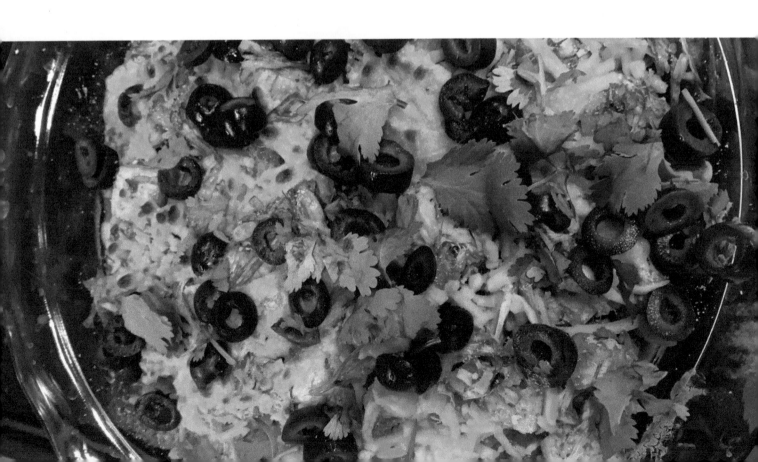

Ratings

Calie - the BBQ sauce and Nacho Cheese sauce together is nacho perfection!

10

Nic – These taste exactly the same as if there was meat on them

10

Fully Loaded Nachos

and remaining ingredients then drizzle with heated Nacho cheese and top with cilantro.

If you are using shredded cheese instead of Nacho cheese...follow these directions.

On a baking sheet covered in parchment paper, layer your chips, top them with your jackfruit, beans and shredded cheese then place in the oven for 10 minutes until the cheese is melted.

Remove from the oven and top with remaining ingredients.

OPTIONAL ADD INS

1. You can easily swap the jackfruit for vegan meat crumbles (but we only use these very occasionally personally), chicken or regular meat for the non-plant based eaters in your house, or just use beans or lentils.
2. Change up the toppings. Jalapenos, sautéed onions, olives (but not for Nic, he hates them) bell peppers are all great nacho toppings.
3. Try swapping traditional chips for a veggie chip. We've made these with kale chips, plantain chips and even zucchini chips thanks to the air fryer. Be creative!

INGREDIENTS

- Chips of your choice - we used Siete grain free chips and blue corn chips
- 1 can of Jackfruit
- BBQ Sauce (see page 132)
- A few tablespoons of beans (refried, black, pinto)
- Handful of romaine, chopped
- 4-5 cherry tomatoes, diced
- ¼ cucumber, diced
- 1 green onion, chopped
- ¼ avocado, diced
- Nacho cheese sauce (see page 134) or vegan cheddar cheese shreds.
- Cilantro

DIRECTIONS

Preheat oven to 425.

In a small sauté pan, heat up your jackfruit with BBQ Sauce. As much sauce as you personally enjoy. But the more sauce the soggier your nachos will be.

In a small saucepan, heat your nacho cheese sauce.

On a baking sheet covered in parchment paper, layer your chips, top them with your jackfruit, beans

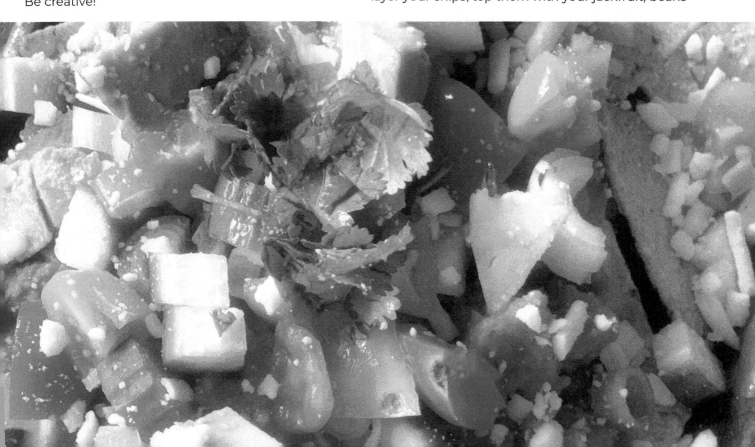

GAME DAY & GIRLS NIGHT

Savory Popcorn

INGREDIENTS

- 1 TBSP olive oil
- ¼ cup organic popcorn seeds
- 2 TBSP unrefined expeller pressed coconut oil (otherwise it will taste like coconut)
- 2 ½ TBSP coconut aminos
- 1- 2 tsp sesame seed oil
- Heavy sprinkling of chili powder
- Heavy sprinkling of smoked paprika
- Light sprinkling of garlic powder
- Light sprinkling of red pepper flakes (optional for more kick)
- Salt

DIRECTIONS

If you've never made stove top popcorn, what rock have you been living under? Go get your kids because they love to watch it pop.

In a medium sauce pan, pour your olive oil and heat over medium heat. Add your popcorn seeds and shake to coat. Put a lid on it and stay with it. You need to watch it closely or it will burn.

Shake occasionally and adjust temperature if you notice the kernels getting overly brown before any start to pop.

Takes about 5 minutes, but once they start popping they'll go quick. When you get down to 3-5 seconds between pops remove from the heat and let it cool while you mix your savory marinade.

In a small bowl, mix the remaining ingredients. You may have to melt your coconut oil because it needs to be liquid or it won't coat the popcorn properly.

Whisk them together and taste test it. Add more seasonings if needed. Pour over your popcorn. Put the lid back on the pot and shake.

OPTIONAL ADD INS

1. Change your savory flavors. Vegan butter with sage leaves and thyme is also absolutely delicious.
2. Toss superfoods into your mix. Chopped nuts. Flax seeds. Pumpkin seeds.
3. Add a little sweetness with dried fruits like goji berries, mulberries, or cranberries.

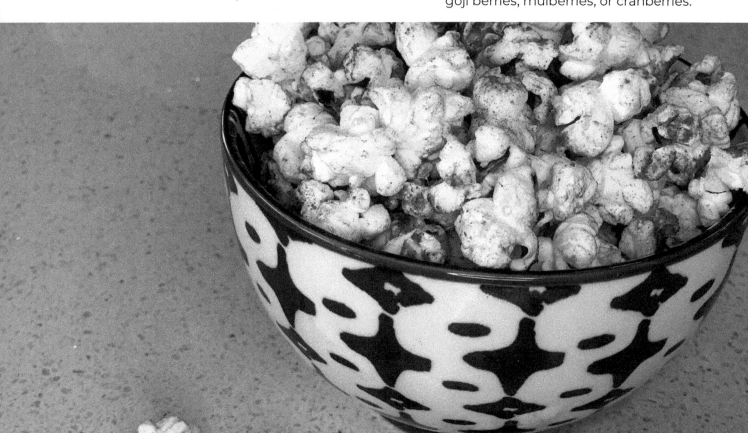

Ratings

Calie - this has been a long time favorite, but I couldn't eat when I realized dairy and [I] don't agree. So naturally we had to recreate it!

 10

Nic – creamy heaven

 10

Pairings

Calie - Platter

Nic – Platter

In a blender add the cashews, nutritional yeast, lemon juice, almond milk, and salt. Blend until very smooth.

Now add the cooked onions/garlic to the blender, plus the spinach, artichokes and a small handful of vegan parmesan. Don't blend it, just use the pulse button a few times so you are left with a chunky texture!

Add additional salt and lemon juice to taste if needed.

Put the mixture into a deep oven dish/pan and bake for around 20 minutes. You will see the mixture turn golden brown and start to bubble.

If you want it really cheesy, top with more parmesan cheese when you remove it from the oven.

Spinach and Artichoke Dip

INGREDIENTS

- 1 ½ cups of cashews (raw and unsalted)
- 1 Yellow onion, chopped
- ¼ cup nutritional yeast
- 1 3/4 cups unsweetened Almond Milk (or any plant-based milk)
- 2 TBSP lemon Juice
- 4 cloves of garlic
- 4 cups of spinach
- 1 Teaspoon of Salt
- 28 Ounces of Artichokes (I used 2 14oz cans)
- Vegan Parmesan (optional but recommended)

DIRECTIONS

Preheat the oven to 420 degrees.

Soak the cashews in boiling water for 5 minutes. Drain

Saute onion and the garlic in 1 TSP of oil for around 3 minutes.

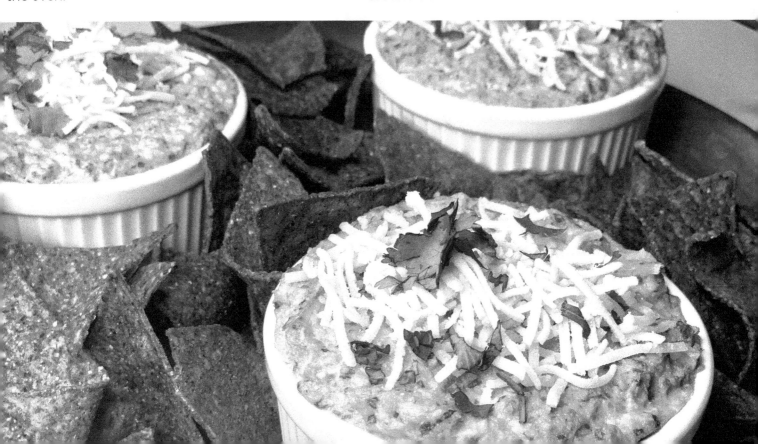

GAME DAY & GIRLS NIGHT

Lemon White Bean Hummus

INGREDIENTS

- 1 14 oz can of cannellini (white) beans
- 2 TBSP Tahini
- 2 TBSP of olive oil
- 1 TBSP of lemon juice
- 2 TBSP of water
- Salt
- 2 tsps of lemon zest
- Optional: A few fresh basil leaves

DIRECTIONS

Toss all of your ingredients into a blender or food processor and pulse until smooth. Taste test to see if you need more salt or want more lemon flavor.

Ratings

Calie - hummus is a staple for me for quick snacks and lemon hummus is my favorite. It really brightens up the flavor. The cannellini beans are a nice change up since we use chickpeas a lot already.

Nic – love hummus wi literally anything

 10

 9

Pairings

Calie - Kebobs

Nic - Kebobs

OPTIONAL ADD INS

1. Red pepper flakes gives it a nice little punch.
2. Thyme or rosemary are great substitutes for the fresh basil.
3. We like to drizzle the top with a little olive oil and some toasted pine nuts when serving it.

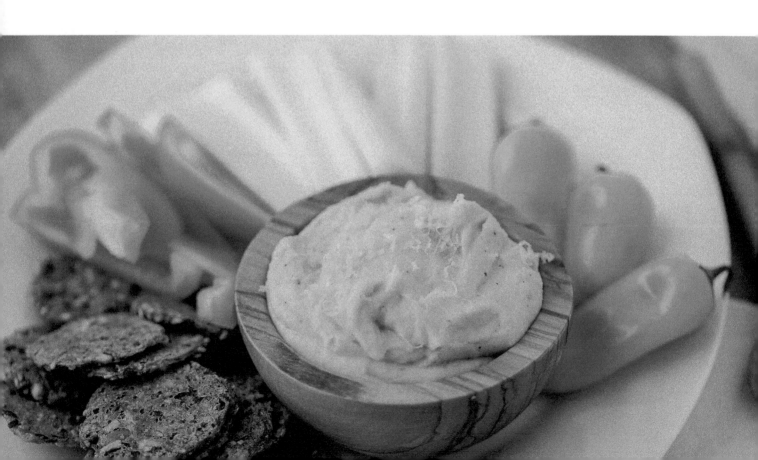

GAME DAY & GIRLS NIGHT

Vegan chilli

DIRECTIONS

In a large soup pan, melt your coconut oil and add garlic and onions. Season with a little salt and pepper and cook for about 3 minutes until onions are translucent. Add your bell peppers and cook another 4-5 minutes stirring often.

Add remaining ingredients. Mix well. Bring to a boil and turn the heat down to low. Simmer for 20 minutes.

OPTIONAL ADD INS

1. Top with a little vegan sour cream. Sprinkle with chopped green onions, cilantro, lime juice.
2. Add shredded vegan cheddar cheese when you serve.
3. Make it heartier for cold winter nights by adding diced, roasted sweet potatoes and a dash of cinnamon.
4. Crumbled tortilla chips or strips.
5. You can always add greens like spinach or swap your onions for something a little different like leeks.

INGREDIENTS

- ¼ yellow onion, diced
- 3 cloves of garlic, thinly sliced
- 1 TBSP coconut oil
- 1 small red pepper, diced
- 1 15 oz can of mixed beans or ½ can each of black beans, pinto beans and kidney beans
- 1 15 oz can of fire roasted diced tomatoes
- 1 10 oz can of diced tomatoes and green chilies (Rotel)
- 1 8 oz can of tomato sauce
- 2 TBSP chili powder
- 2 tsp of cumin
- 2 tsp of paprika
- 1 tsp of oregano
- ¼ tsp of red pepper flakes
- Salt
- Black Pepper

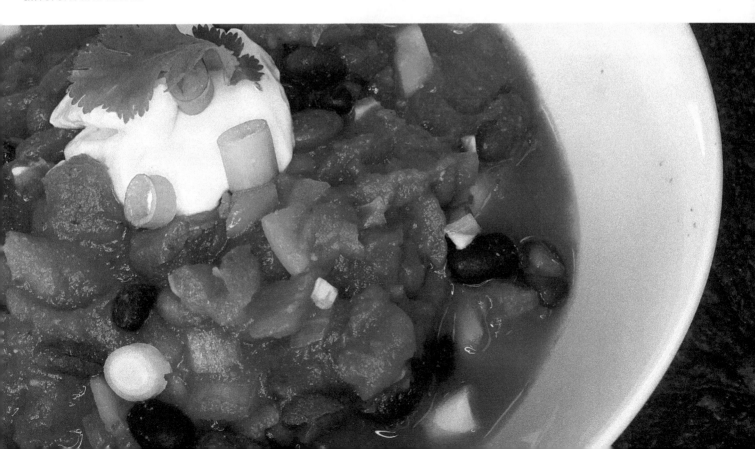

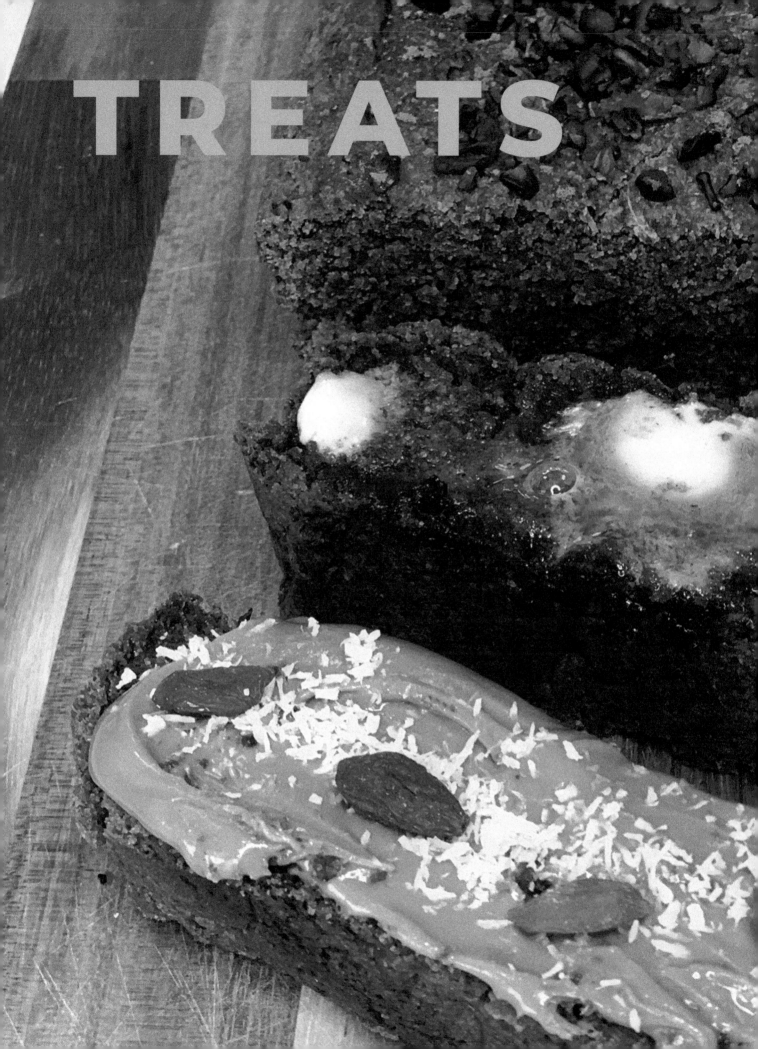

TREATS

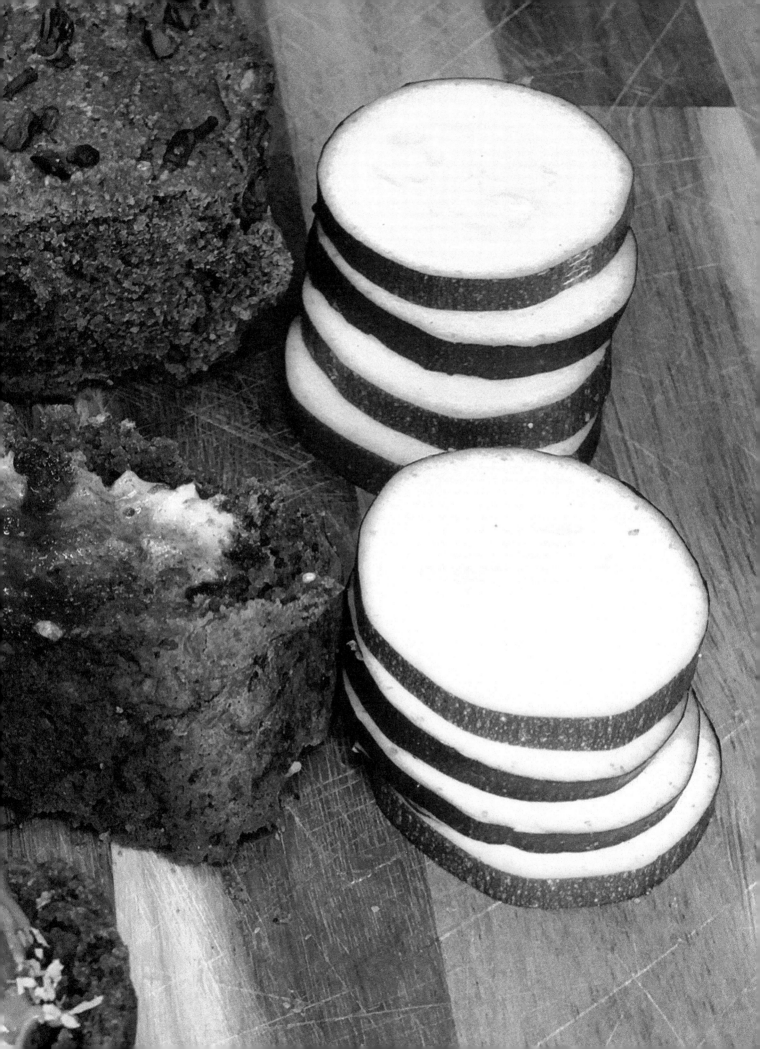

TREATS

SuperFood Fudge

INGREDIENTS

- 12 pitted medjool dates soaked in hot water for 3-5 minutes and draine
- ½ cup Vegan Chocolate Protein or Collagen powder or unsweetened cocoa powder
- 4 Tablespoons of coconut oil
- 1 Tablespoon of coconut butter
- ¼ tsp vanilla extract
- ¼ tsp salt
- 1 tsp of maca powder
- ¼ tsp cinnamon
- 1/8 tsp nutmeg
- Unsweetened almond butter
- Hemp hearts
- Mulberries
- Goji berries
- Unsweetened shredded coconut

DIRECTIONS

Line a small glass baking dish or loaf pan with parchment paper so you can easily lift the fudge out when it's chilled.

In a blender, combine the dates, cocoa powder, coconut oil, coconut butter, vanilla extract, salt, maca powder, cinnamon and nutmeg. Blend until well combined and creamy. You might need to scrape down the sides and mix it as you go.

Pour into your baking dish and press it flat and even with a spatula. Drizzle with unsweetened almond butter and sprinkle the top with hemp hearts, coconut flakes, mulberries and goji berries. Sprinkle with salt. Cover with parchment paper and chill 2-4 hours.

OPTIONAL ADD INS

1. Fold any combo of dried or frozen fruit into your batter after you take it out of the blender. Crushed plantain chips are great sprinkled on top.
2. Add chopped nuts, cacao nibs or dark chocolate chips or peanut butter chips to the batter after you blend it.
3. Sprinkle matcha powder on top.
4. Swap the almond butter drizzle for the caramel sauce used in the turtles.

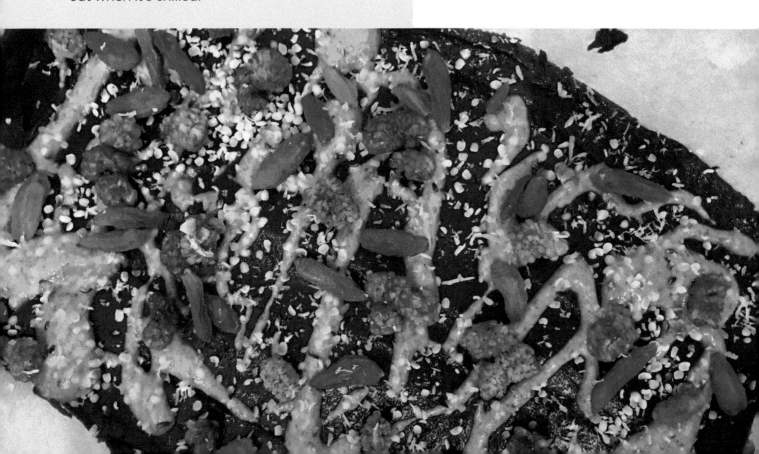

Nic – can I rate this more than a 10?

10

...lie - Nic and I got into a ...on fight trying to get the ...t bite of this one! Sadly, he won...bully!

10

TREATS

Cookies and Ice Cream

INGREDIENTS

- Sweet Loren's take & bake cookies (we prefer chocolate chip)
- NadaMoo Lotta Mint Chip ice cream

DIRECTIONS

It's treat night, so treat yourself to a night off of cooking and baking with the help of these amazing, super clean (for treats) and easy to find in most stores, plant-based brands that we absolutely love!

Bake 2 cookies per person according to the package directions. Don't bake more or you'll eat them all! They are literally the best chocolate chip cookies. If Calie is around, hide them, because she eats the dough raw (which is perfectly safe since these are plant-based!) and there will be none left for anyone else.

Let the cookies cool after you take them out of the oven and add a scoop of NadaMoo Lotta Mint Chip ice cream.

If you really want to have fun with it...roll the edges in cacao nibs for a fancy, mouthwatering, but super easy ice cream sandwich.

OPTIONAL ADD INS

1. Sweet Loren's also has a double chocolate chip cookie if you want to go heavy on the chocolate or a sugar cookie for a simpler option.
2. Change the ice cream flavor.
3. Roll the sides in chopped nuts, dye free sprinkles, or add coconut whip cream to the top.

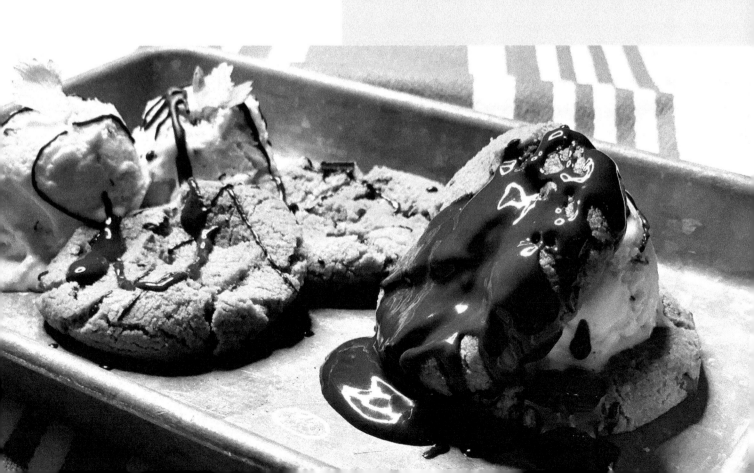

TREATS

Superfood Chocolate Clusters

CENTER INGREDIENTS

- Pistachios
- Cashews
- Walnuts
- Sunflower seeds
- Chia seeds
- Unsweetened almond butter
- Salt

CHOCOLATE INGREDIENTS

- ¼ cup of cacao nibs or vegan dark chocolate (we love the HU bars for these)
- 1 TBSP of coconut oil

CARAMEL INGREDIENTS

- 1 can of sweetened condensed coconut milk (unopened)

DIRECTIONS

Based on how many you want to make, toss some nuts and seeds into a bowl and sprinkle with salt. Add about 1 TBSP almond butter per cluster you are planning to make. Mix together

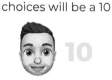
with your hands and roll into individual balls. Lay them out on a baking sheet covered in parchment paper and press flat.

In a small sauce pan, add coconut oil and chocolate and melt over low heat stirring continuously. You want it to be thick enough that it won't run everywhere so adjust as needed by adding more chocolate or even a tiny bit of gluten-free flour to the mix if you need to thicken it a little bit. Pour the chocolate over each cluster until it's completely covered.

Place the pan in the freezer to set.

While the chocolate is setting, place your unopened can of condensed coconut milk in a small sauce pan and cover it completely with water. Bring it to a low boil and boil for 2 hours...refilling the water as needed so it stays covered the whole time.

Remove it from the water after 2 hours and let the can cool completely before opening it. When your caramel sauce is ready, remove the clusters from the freezer and drizzle with caramel sauce. Sprinkle tops with a little more salt and store in the fridge or eat immediately.

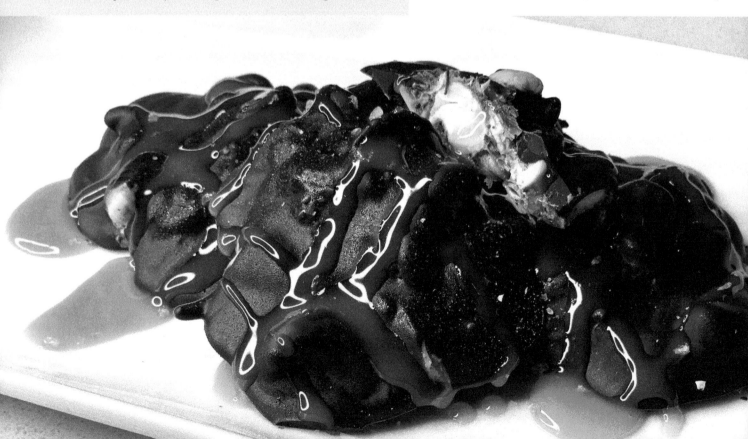

Peanut Butter Whiskey

Ratings

Calie - so nice! Kill the cocktail and sweet craving in one delicious drink. Nutmeg would be good on top too.

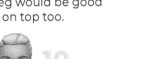

10

Nic – Perfect late night movie drink

10

INGREDIENTS

- Screwball Peanut Butter Whiskey
- Almond Milk or Coconut Milk
- Cinnamon
- Dark chocolate shavings
- Ice

DIRECTIONS

In a mason jar, or glass of your choice, add ice, one shot of peanut butter whiskey and then fill to the top with unsweetened almond milk. Sprinkle with cinnamon and dark chocolate shavings and sip your dessert. Try not to chug it. It's like a grown up milkshake and you'll get a different kind of brain freeze if you drink it too fast.

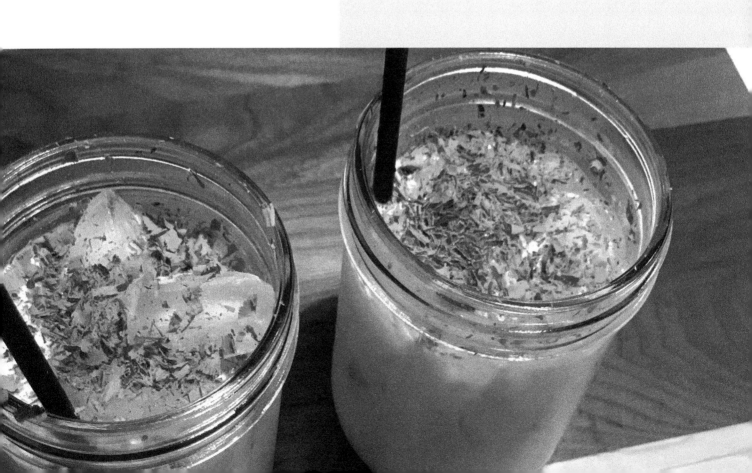

TREATS

Strawberry Lemonade Gut Goodies

INGREDIENTS

- 1/2 cup of vegan vanilla protein powder
- 1/2 cup of green banana flour
- 1/2 cup of unsweetened almond butter
- 1/4 cup of orange blossom honey
- 1 TBSP crushed freeze dried strawberries
- 1 TBSP of watermelon BCAA+G recover powder or l-glutamine powder
- 1/4 tsp of lemon extract
- maca powder for dusting

Ratings

Calie - I'm a chocolate girl, which is the only reason these aren't a 10. My friends ask me to make these for every summer party.

 8

Nic – surprised when Calie made these! So good

 9

DIRECTIONS

Combine all the ingredients in a bowl and mix together until it forms a soft dough like texture. Use a tablespoon to scoop out serving and roll between your hands into a ball. Roll in maca powder and freeze for 20-30 minutes for best taste and texture. Store in the fridge for up to 5 days or in the freezer until they're gone.

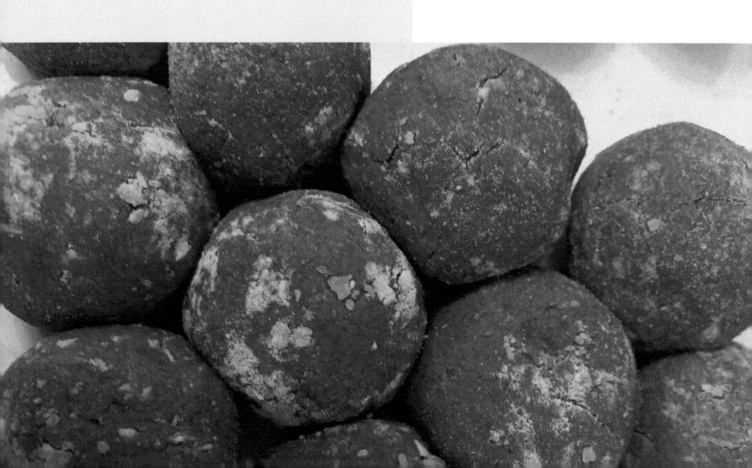

alie - if you don't make
his...you're missing out!

 10

Nic – nice texture..yes ill use
that word...moist!

 8

TREATS

Zucchini Bread

In a large bowl mix your dry ingredients.

In a small bowl, mix your wet ingredients minus the zucchini.

Pour the wet mixture into the dry mix and combine with a spatula or your hands. It will seem dry at first. Keep working it. You'll get more of a clumpy dough than a batter.

Fold in your zucchini then press the mixture into your loaf pan.

Top with sprinkle of cacao nibs.

Bake for 50 minutes, until a toothpick inserted comes out clean.

Allow it to cool completely before cutting or it will fall apart.

OPTIONAL ADD INS

1. You can add walnuts, dried fruit, chia seeds or any other super foods or nuts of your choice.
2. Swap the zucchini for shredded carrots and add ¼ tsp of cinnamon
3. Top your finished bread with vegan butter, nut butter and fresh fruit like blueberries or bananas, drizzle of honey, or butter and honey mixed. Yum!

DRY INGREDIENTS

- 1 cup of banana flour
- 1 cup of fine almond flour
- ½ tsp baking soda
- 1 tsp baking powder
- ½ tsp of salt
- 1 tsp of cinnamon
- ¼ tsp of nutmeg
- Topping: cacao nibs (optional)

WET INGREDIENTS

- ¼ cup of melted coconut oil
- 2 TBSP of olive oil
- ¼ cup of maple syrup
- ¼ cup unsweetened almond butter
- 1 ½ flax eggs (4 ½ tsp of flax + ¼ cup of water - let it sit while you mix the rest of your ingredients.
- 1 tsp of vanilla extract
- 1 cup of grated zucchini (fold in at the end)

DIRECTIONS

Preheat oven to 325 degrees. Spray a loaf pan with a little coconut oil cooking spray then line with parchment paper.

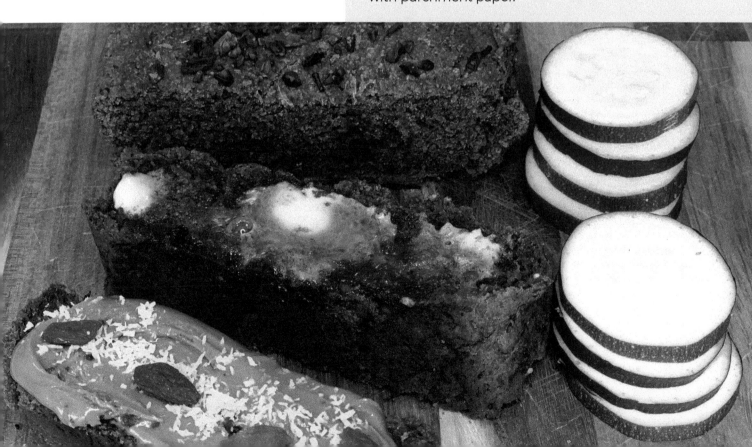

SAUCES

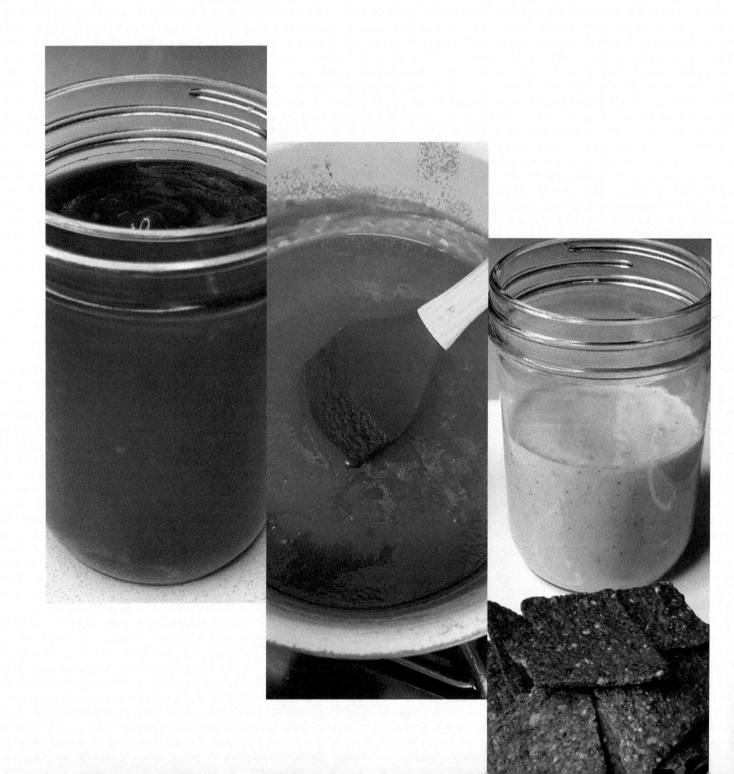

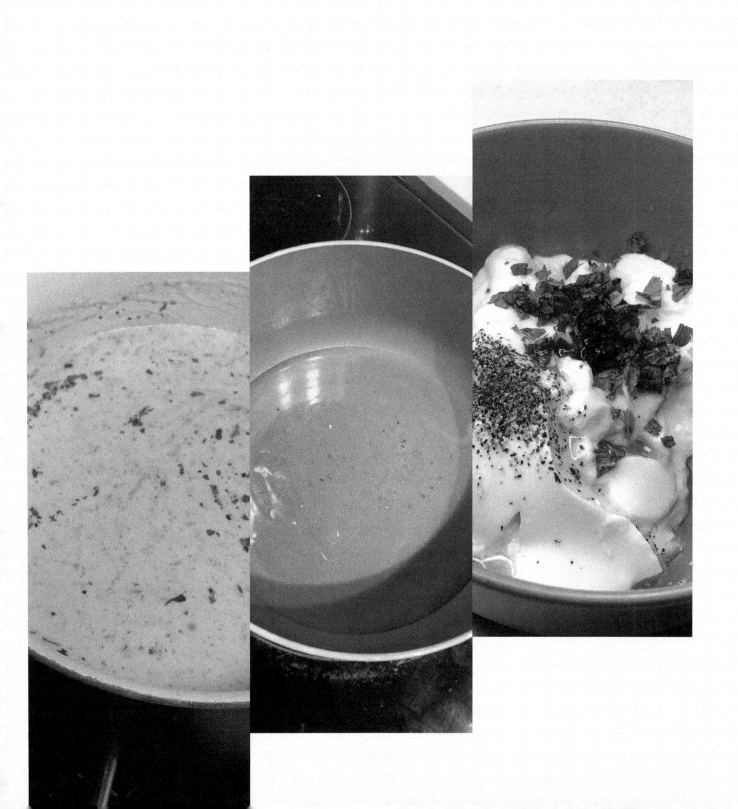

SAUCES

BBQ Sauce

INGREDIENTS

- 2 cups of ketchup (you can use our smoky ketchup or store bought but no sugar added)
- ¼ cup of pure grade maple syrup
- ¼ cup of apple cider vinegar
- 1 TBSP of coconut aminos
- 1 TBSP of worcestershire sauce plus a little
- 2 tsps of sriracha or cholula hot sauce

Ratings

Calie - so much flavor!

9

Nic – so good on prett much anything!

9

Pairings

Calie - Tricolored fries

Nic – Tofu Nuggests

DIRECTIONS

Combine all of the Ingredients in a small sauce pan and cook over low heat stirring the whole time for about 5 minutes.

Allow it to cool. Transfer to a storage container and store in the fridge for up to a week.

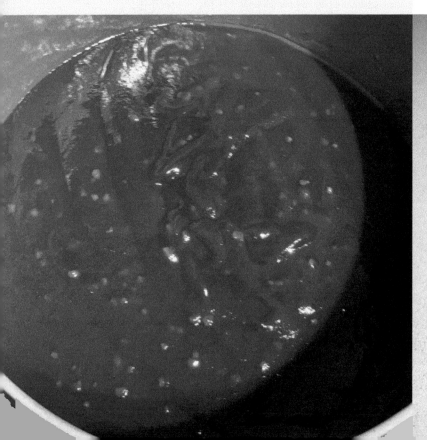

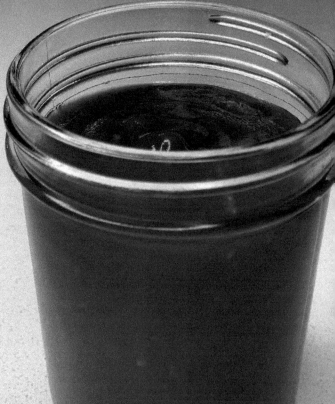

Ratings

Pairings

Calie - Lentil meatloaf   Nic - Anything

DIRECTIONS

Throw it all in a small saucepan. Whisk and heat until you get a slow rolling boil over medium heat. Turn it off. Let it sit for about 30 minutes to thicken and you're ready to dip!

SAUCES

Smokey Ketchup

INGREDIENTS

- 16 oz can of tomato paste
- 5 TBSP dark pure grade maple syrup
- ¾ cup of water
- ¼ cup of apple cider vinegar
- 1 tsp garlic powder
- 1 tsp smoked paprika
- ¼ tsp cinnamon
- Salt to taste
- 1 TBSP Stone Ground Mustard or Dijon Mustard

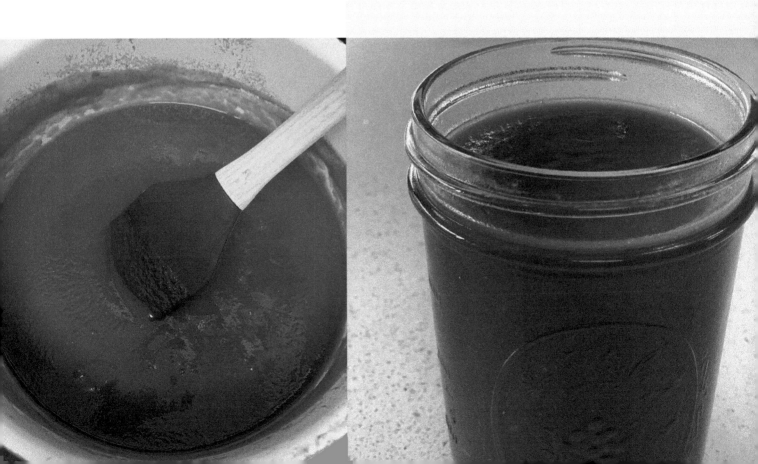

SAUCES

Nacho Cheese Dip

INGREDIENTS

- 1 ¼ cups of soaked raw cashews
- 1 TBSP lemon juice
- ¼ cup nutritional yeast
- 2 oz canned diced green chillies
- 1 TBSP chilli powder
- 3 tsp cumin
- 1 ½ tsp paprika
- ¼ tsp each oregano, garlic powder, onion powder
- 1 tsp each salt and black pepper
- ¼ tsp red pepper flakes
- 2 cups vegetable broth

DIRECTIONS

Soak your cashews completely covered in water for at least 3 hours. Drain and rinse them.

Place all of your Ingredients in a blender and blend on high for at least 30 seconds until smooth.

Ratings

Calie - this sauce is so versatile and my boys request it. They have no idea it doesn't have cheese in it, hahahaha! Well, they do now ;)

Nic – again, dump it on anything you want. Ooooo dip a burger in it

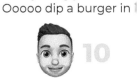

9

10

Pairings

Calie - Loaded Nachos

Nic – I dump this on everything

Pour into a medium sauce pan and heat over medium heat for 3-5 minutes stirring continuously until it thickens.

Store in the fridge.

OPTIONAL ADD INS

1. You can add taco seasoned lentils or even ground chicken or turkey if you aren't trying to be totally plant-based.
2. Add a little jalapeno to really spice it up.
3. Add ¼ of a red bell pepper to the blender to give it a little more spice and that "yellow" nacho cheese color.

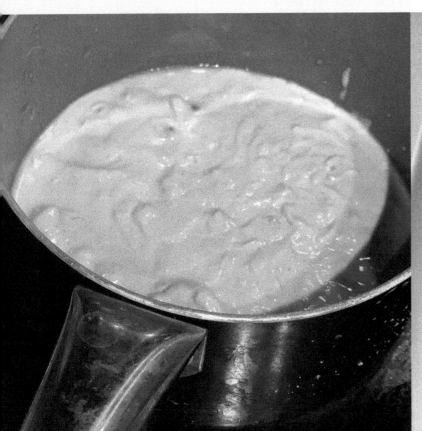

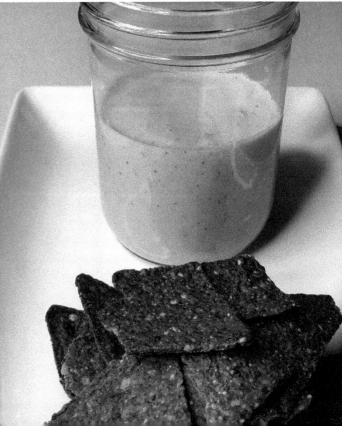

Ratings

Pairings

Calie - Butternut squash
pasta

Nic – Butternut squash
pasta

DIRECTIONS

Rinse and drain the almonds. Put your almonds, milk, water, garlic, salt and nutritional yeast in a blender and blend until smooth. At least 30 seconds.

In a medium saucepan, melt your butter and add the flour. Stir continuously for about 2 minutes. Slowly pour the almond mixture into the pan stirring continuously to combine and prevent sticking and burning.

Add the black pepper and parsley and continuing heating over medium heat stirring continuously for about 5 minutes until the sauce thickens.

Remove from heat and let it cool. Store in the fridge.

SAUCES

Garlic Parmesan Cream Sauce

INGREDIENTS

- 1 cup of raw almonds soaked in water for 2-3 hours
- 1 cup of unsweetened almond milk
- 1 cup of water
- 3 cloves of garlic, peeled
- Salt to taste (we use about ¼ tsp otherwise it's salty)
- ¼ cup nutritional yeast
- 2 TBSP vegan butter
- 3 TBSP gluten-free all purpose flour (we used Cup 4 Cup)
- 1 tsp of black pepper...and a little bit more
- 1 TBSP dried parsley

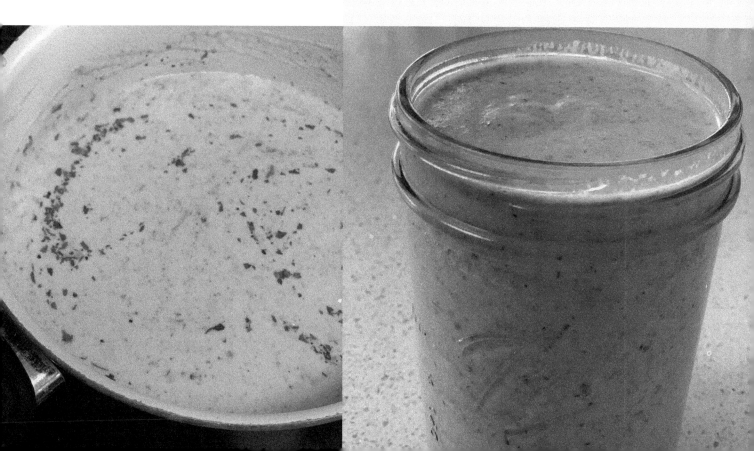

SAUCES

Peanut Sauce

INGREDIENTS

- 2 TBSP grated ginger
- 4 cloves of garlic
- 4 TBSP raw unsalted peanut butter
- 2 TBSP raw honey
- 3 TBSP Bragg's Liquid Aminos
- Crushed red pepper flakes
- Salt

Ratings

Calie - this is one of my go to sauces every week. I love making peanut stir fries with it!

 9

Nic – up there with my fa of all time

 10

Pairings

Calie - Spring rolls   Nic - Anything

DIRECTIONS

Combine all of the Ingredients in a large mixing bowl. Whisk until well combined. This is amazing on veggies, rice dishes grilled tofu, tempeh and as a dip for spring rolls.

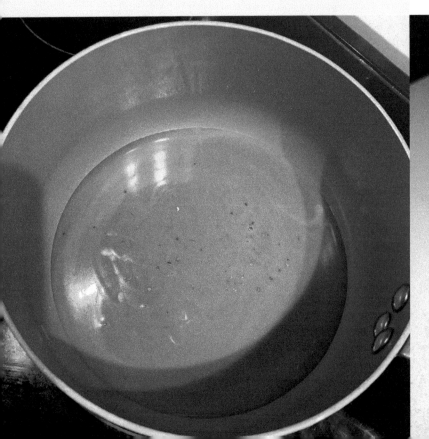

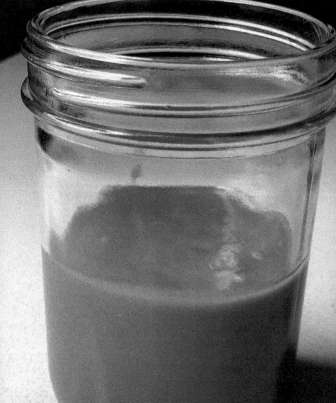

Ratings

Calie - lick the bowl good

 10

Nic – so refreshing

 10

Pairings

Calie - Platter

Nic - Kabobs

DIRECTIONS

Just go ahead and make a double batch. You're gonna need it. This is freaking delicious on everything! And ridiculously easy.

Step 1. Mix all the Ingredients together in a bowl.

Step 2. Stick in fridge for 20 mins

No really, that's it.

Plant-based living is SOOO HARD! I don't have time...said no one whoever really gave it a shot.

Mint Yogurt Dressing

INGREDIENTS

- 1 Cup of Plant-Based Almond Yogurt
  (You can also use Soy or Coconut Yogurt)
- 2 TBSP Olive Oil
- 4 TBSP Lemon Juice
- 4 Cloves of finely chopped Garlic
- 3 TBSP Fresh Mint chopped
- 1 TSP Salt
- ½ TSP Pepper

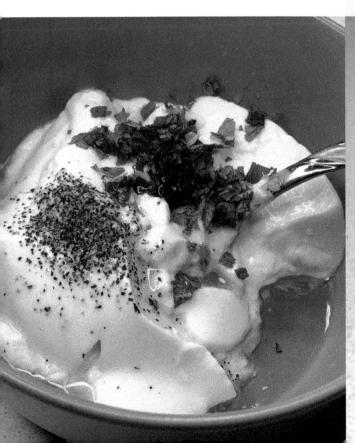

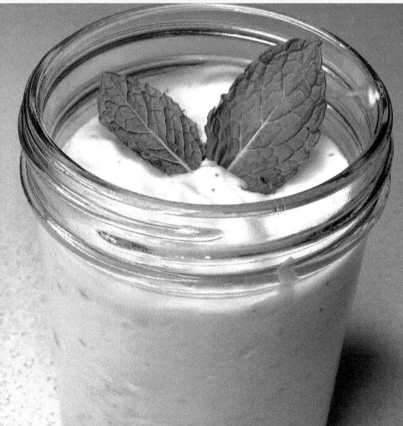

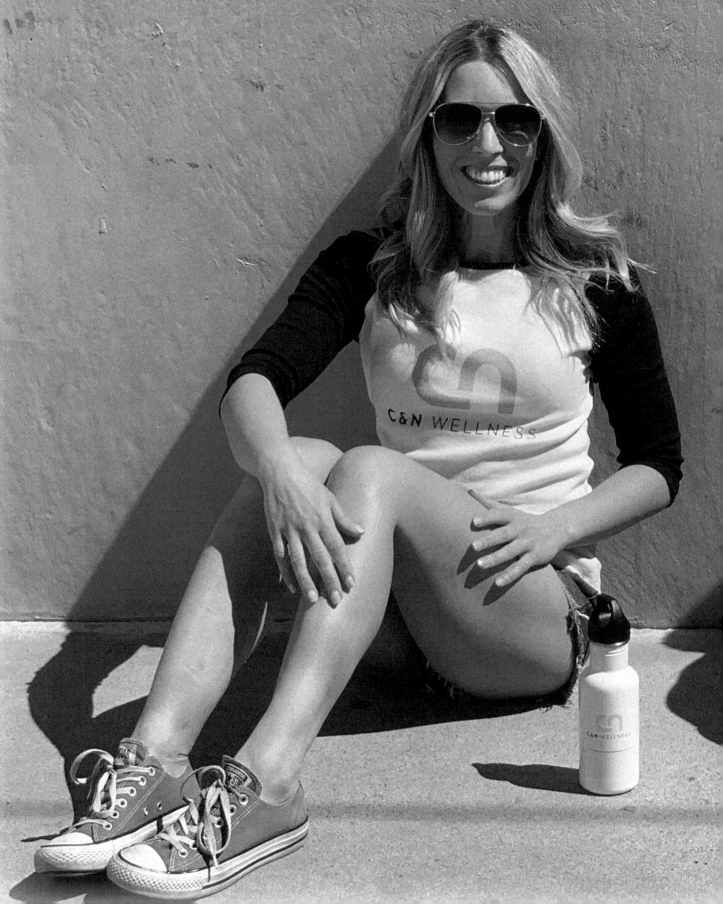

CALIE

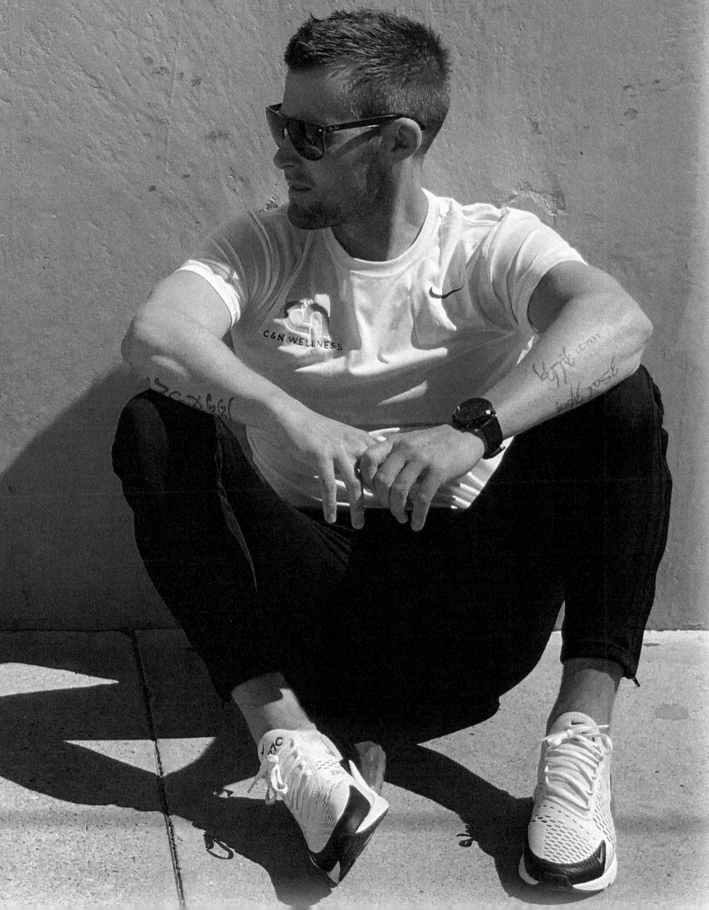

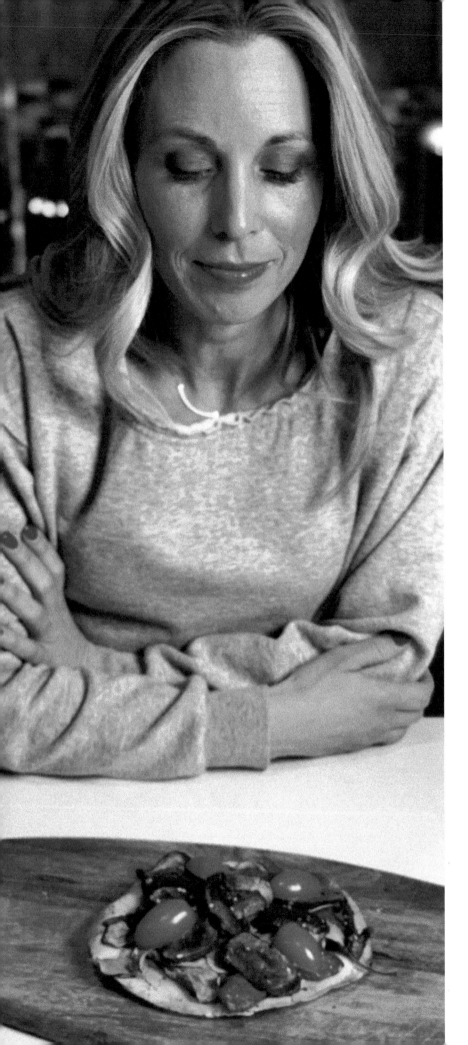

BBQ Thin Crust Pizza

INGREDIENTS

- 2 Gluten-Free Brown Rice Wraps
- Vegan Mozzarella Cheese
- Smoky Tempeh
- Eggplant, thinly sliced
- Zucchini, thinly sliced
- Onion, thinly sliced
- Cherry Tomatoes, halved
- Buffalo Sauce
- Jalapenos, thinly sliced
- Oregano
- Salt
- Black Pepper

DIRECTIONS

1. Preheat oven to 375.
2. Lay one wrap on a baking sheet and layer with mozzarella cheese and a drizzle of buffalo sauce. I like Tessamae's Mild Buffalo Sauce. Top it with your second wrap and drizzle that one with buffalo sauce too.
3. Layer your remaining ingredients on top and sprinkle with a little oregano, salt and black pepper.
4. Place it in the oven and bake for about 15-20 minutes until warmed through and cheese is melted.
5. Drizzle with a little more buffalo sauce if you love it as much as I do!
6. Cut it in half and pretend you're not going to eat the whole thing in one sitting!

Ratings

Calie - I literally dream about this pizza!

 10

Nic – love a thin crust. Well done Calie on this.

 10

Meat Lovers Pizza

INGREDIENTS

- Vegan Nan Bread
- Garlic Parmesan Sauce
- Plant Based "Ground Beef"
- Plant Based Sausage
- Mushrooms, thinly sliced
- Spinach
- Cherry Tomatoes, halved
- Vegan Cheddar & Mozzarella cheese mix

DIRECTIONS

1. Preheat oven to 400.
2. Throw all ingredients into a pan with olive oil and saute for around 10 minutes.
3. Lay your bread on a baking sheet, spread a generous amount of parmesan garlic sauce on it. Transfer sauteed ingredients on top. Cover with grated vegan cheese.
4. Place it in the oven and bake for about 10 minutes until warmed through and cheese is melted.
5. Drizzle with a little more garlic parmesan sauce and you're done!
6. Eat it, feel happy, satisfied and a million times more energized and healthy than you would after greasy delivery.

Ratings

ie - I was disappointed. xpected bold "meaty" vors, but the fake meat oesn't do it for me. I'll ick to my veggie pizza.

5

Nic - Calie is a lunatic!

10

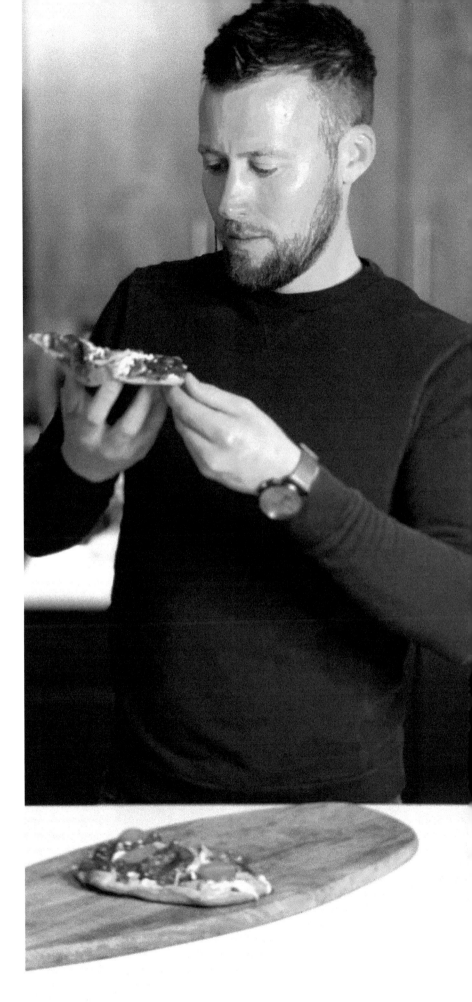

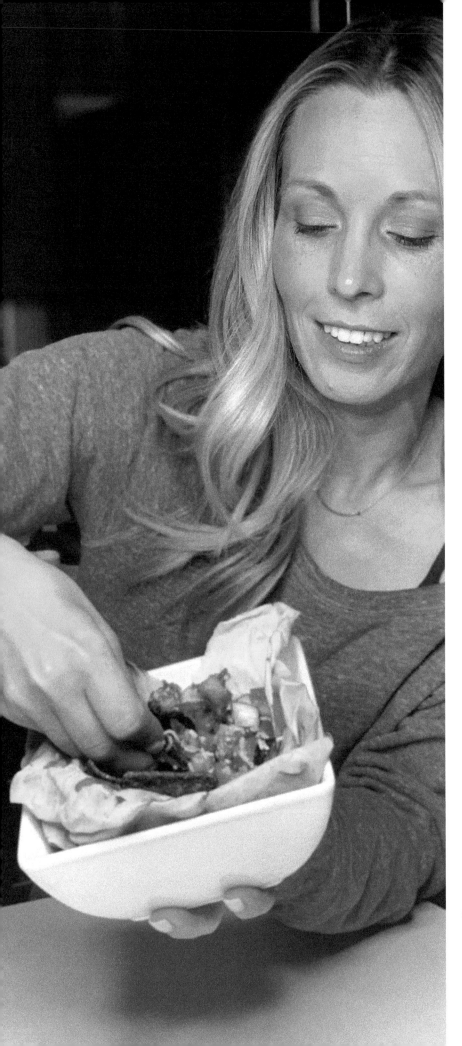

Eggplant Taco Bowl

INGREDIENTS

- Eggplant, diced
- Mushrooms, thinly sliced
- Red onion, thinly sliced
- 1 clove of garlic, thinly sliced
- Cherry tomatoes, halved
- ¼ cucumber, diced
- Cilantro
- 2 Butter lettuce leaves
- Sriracha sauce
- Chili powder
- Cumin
- Smoked paprika
- Oregano
- Garlic powder
- Onion powder
- Red pepper flakes
- Olive oil

DIRECTIONS

1. In a saute pan, drizzle olive oil and toss in all of your veggies except for the cucumbers, tomatoes and butter lettuce leaves.
2. Sprinkle heavily with chili powder, cumin and smoked paprika and lightly with oregano, garlic powder, onion powder and red pepper flakes.
3. Saute over medium heat for about 10-12 minutes until the eggplant is cooked through and soft.
4. Place your butter lettuce leaves in a bowl. Fill with your taco filling. Sprinkle with vegan cheddar cheese and top with cucumber, tomatoes and cilantro. Drizzle with a little Sriracha sauce and be shocked that you don't miss the traditional shell.

Ratings

Calie - because I'm competitive and Nic's was more creative and looked prettier. But honestly, the traditional taco seasoning mixed with this veggie combo makes a seriously solid dish.

 9

Nic – yeah definitely alternative. But I love crunch so give me taco shells any day

 8

Curry Chicken Tacos

INGREDIENTS

- Plant Based Chicken
- Curry Powder
- Refried beans
- Salt
- Romaine, chopped
- Tomatoes, diced
- Vegan cheddar cheese
- Blue Corn Taco Shells
- Buffalo Sauce

DIRECTIONS

1. In a small saute pan, drizzle a little olive oil and toss in your plant-based chicken. Season heavily with curry seasoning mix, salt and pepper.
2. While that's warming, open a can of refried beans and scoop a few tablespoons into a small saucepan and warm them through.
3. Assemble ingredients in your taco shells and drizzle with Buffalo Sauce or Hot Sauce of your choice.
4. Smile (and gloat a little) because this is a winning dish!

Ratings

ie - damn it....that curry icken was such a good idea! He got me!

 9

Nic - I'm taking a bow

 10

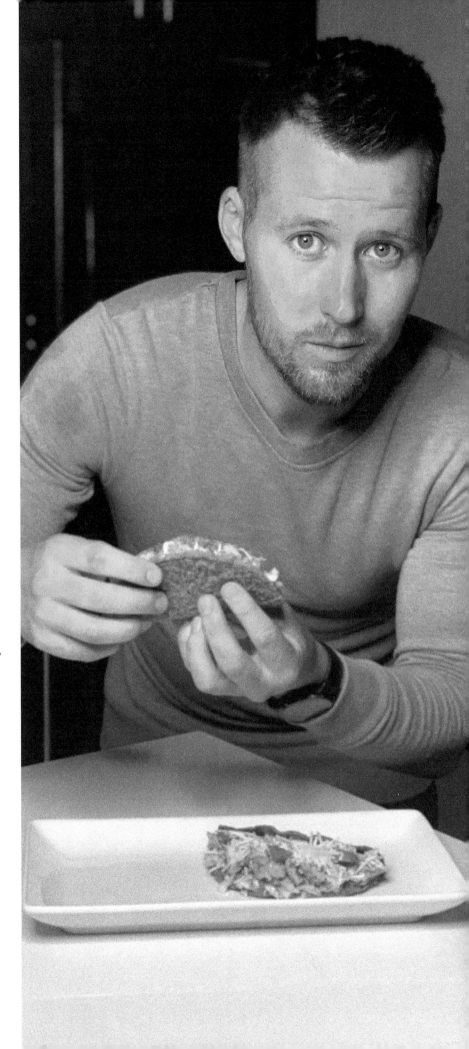

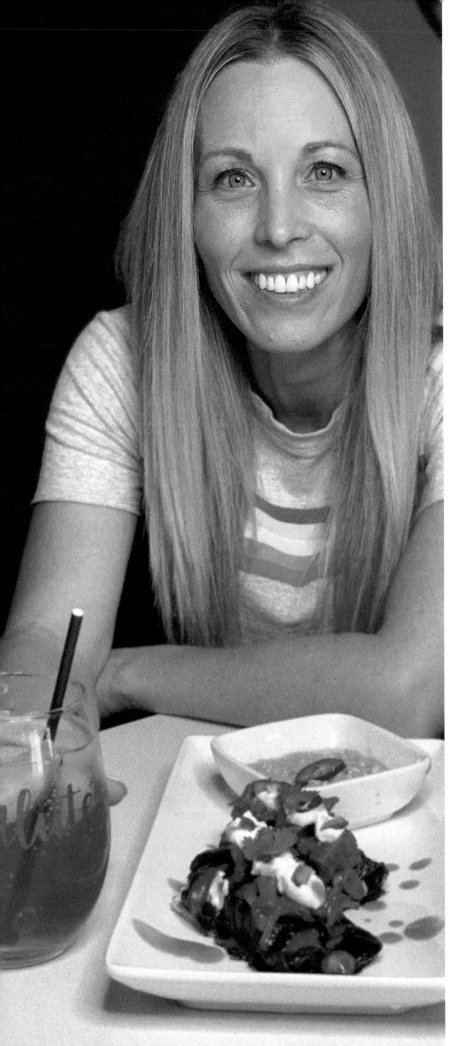

Spicy BBQ Jackfruit Roll

INGREDIENTS

- 1 Nori roll
- Jasmine rice
- Vegan cream cheese
- Thinly sliced cucumber
- Thinly sliced carrots
- Bamboo sprouts
- 1 piece of smoky tempeh bacon
- BBQ jackfruit
- Vegan mayo
- Buffalo sauce
- Avocado
- Jalapeno
- Cilantro

DIRECTIONS

1. Preheat oven to 375.
2. Cook your jasmine rice. We used a microwave bag for convenience.
3. Lay out your nori wrap. Place a thin layer of rice on the far left edge. Place cucumber, carrot and bamboo slices along the edge in a very thin layer. Put a thin layer of vegan cream cheese next to your veggies and then add your tempeh bacon slice.
4. Gently roll your nori wrap closed, tucking it to make it tight. Lay BBQ jackfruit on top and drizzle with buffalo sauce then bake for 10 minutes.
5. While your roll is baking mix vegan mayo with buffalo sauce and ⅛ of an avocado. Top with a slice of jalapeno
6. Cut your baked roll into halves, drizzle with buffalo sauce and top with a little bit of vegan mayo, diced jalapeno and cilantro leaves.
7. Admit that Nic's roll looks so much more appetizing, but celebrate the fact that yours wins for flavor!

Ratings

Calie - but honestly... it's a 10!

Nic – Fuck Sake. Ye

10   10

Crispy Baked Avocado Roll

INGREDIENTS

- 1 Nori wrap
- 2 TBSP jasmine rice
- Thinly sliced carrots
- Thinly sliced cucumber
- Vegan cream cheese
- Thinly sliced avocado
- Bamboo sprouts
- Vegan crab meat
- Vegan mayo
- Buffalo sauce
- Wakami

DIRECTIONS

1. Preheat oven to 375.
2. Cook your jasmine rice. We used a microwave bag for convenience.
3. Lay out your nori wrap. Place a thin layer of rice on the far left edge. Place cucumber, carrot and bamboo slices along the edge in a very thin layer. Put a thin layer of vegan cream cheese next to your veggies and top it with thinly sliced avocado.
4. Gently roll your nori wrap closed, tucking it gently to make it tight. Lay vegan crab meat on top and bake for 10 minutes.
5. While your roll is baking mix vegan mayo with buffalo sauce to taste.
6. Cut your baked roll into 4 pieces, drizzle with buffalo mayo and top with wakame bits.
7. Assume your roll is better than Calie's and prepare to be wrong ;)

Ratings

Calie – a reluctant 9 for flavor and 10 for presentation. I'd order this at a sushi restaurant!

 9

Nic – I'm fucking proud of this one

 10

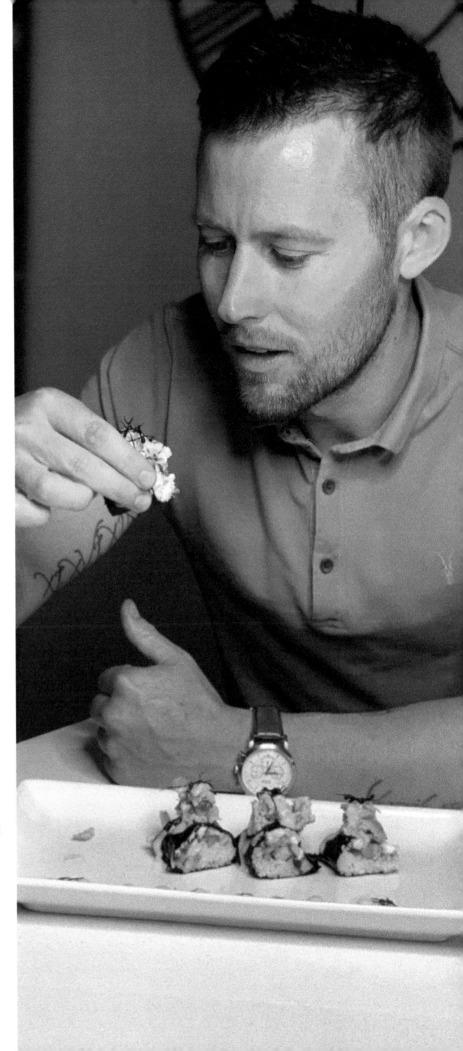

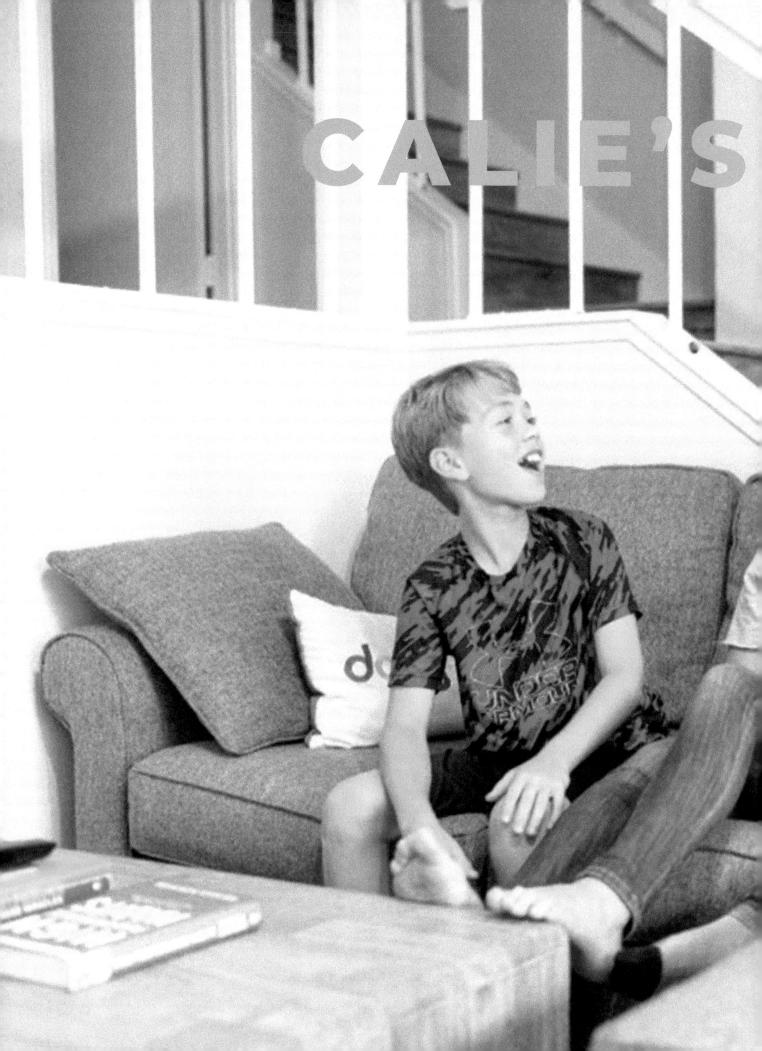

FAVORITES

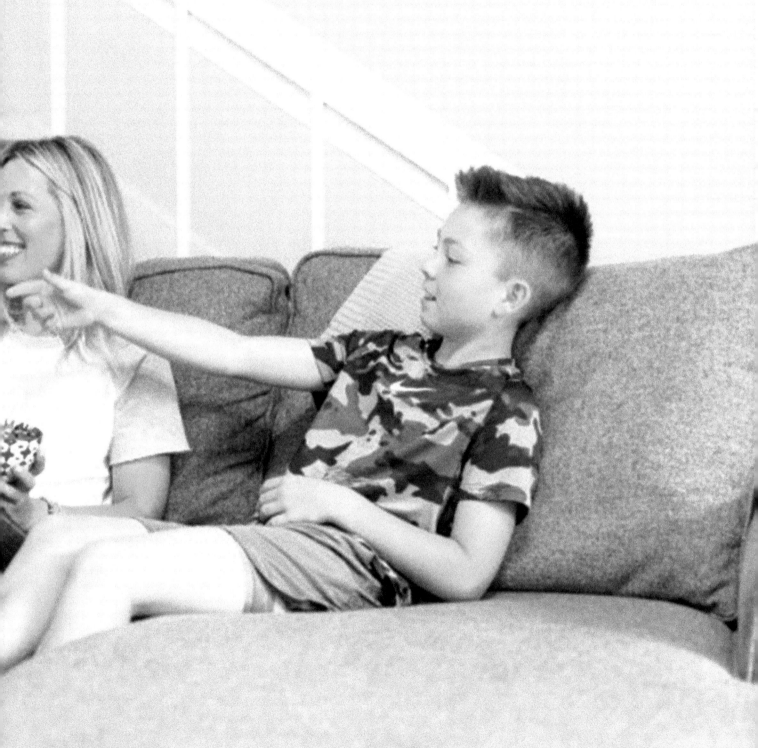

Lasagna

INGREDIENTS

- 1 large Eggplant
- 1 portobello mushroom, diced 10-12 cherry tomatoes or 3-4 romas, diced
- ¼ yellow onion
- 2 cloves of garlic
- Vegan parmesan or mozzarella
- Olive oil
- Salt
- Black pepper
- Garlic powder
- Basil
- Oregano
- Parsley

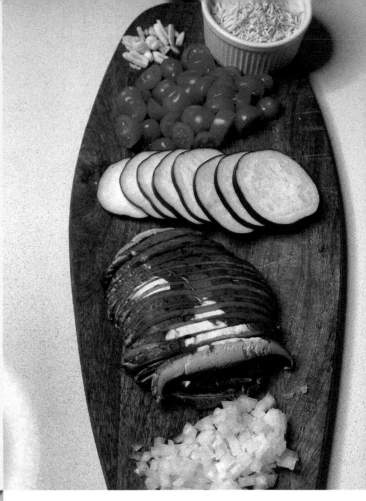

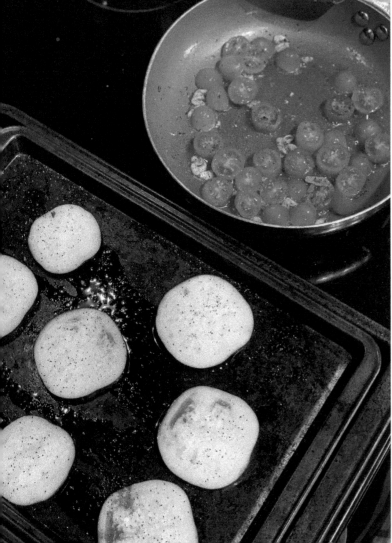

DIRECTIONS

1. Preheat oven to 400 degrees.
2. Slice your eggplant into ¼ inch thin sheets or rounds depending on your pan. Drizzle with olive oil and sprinkle with salt and pepper. Bake for 25 minutes.
3. While your eggplant is baking prepare your mushroom mince by placing a drizzle of olive oil in a saute pan. Add your chopped onion and sprinkle with salt and pepper. Cook for 3 minutes until translucent then add your mushrooms. Cook for another 5-7 minutes. Set aside.
4. Prepare your sauce. Put about ¼ cup of olive oil in a saute pan. Toss in your garlic and cook for about 2 minutes stirring frequently. Add your diced tomatoes and sprinkle heavily with basil, a little oregano, salt and pepper. Cook until tomatoes are totally wilted about 5-7 minutes. Place mix in blender and puree.

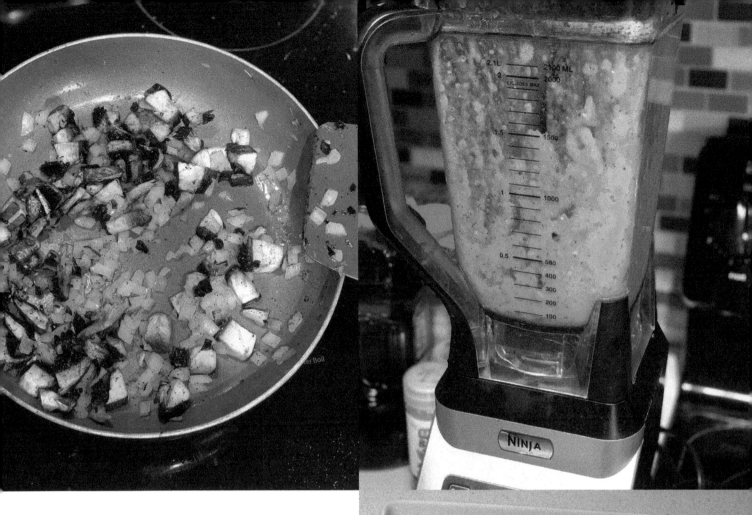

5. Remove eggplant from the oven and layer in your baking dish. Eggplant, mushroom mince, tomato sauce, cheese, eggplant, tomato sauce, cheese.

6. Place the dish back in the oven for about 10 minutes until cheese melts and your sauce bubbles.

7. Top with fresh parsley or basil and enjoy!

Ratings

Calie - I'd order this at a restaurant over and over again.

Nic – one of my top dishes from this book.

 9

 10

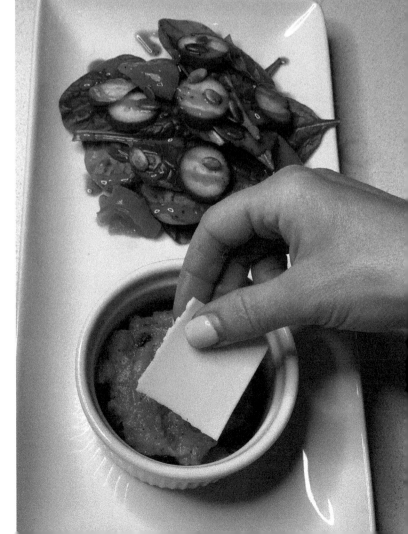

Fries Two Ways With Smoked Ketchup

TRICOLOR FRIES INGREDIENTS

- Purple sweet potato
- Orange sweet potato
- White potato
- Olive oil
- Salt
- Black pepper

DIRECTIONS

Cut your potatoes into wedges. Place them in a large saucepan, cover with water and sprinkle with salt. (Note: We boil the purple potatoes in a separate pan because they turn everything else dark purple. But this is just for aesthetics. Don't waste your time or pan if you're just going for taste.) Bring to a boil, turn the heat down to medium and simmer for 15 minutes.

Drain the potatoes and drizzle with a tiny bit of olive oil massaging it all over the fries. Sprinkle with salt and pepper and transfer to air fryer in a single layer. Fry at 400 degrees for 8 minutes, flip and fry an additional 8 minutes. Repeat until all of your potato wedges are done.

Serve with smoked ketchup or vegan ranch.

Loaded Turnip Fries

INGREDIENTS

- 1 large turnip cut into fry shaped wedges
- 2-3 slices of smoky tempeh bacon
- 2-3 cherry tomatoes
- 1 green onion
- Cilantro
- Sour cream
- Buffalo sauce
- Salt
- Black pepper
- Garlic powder

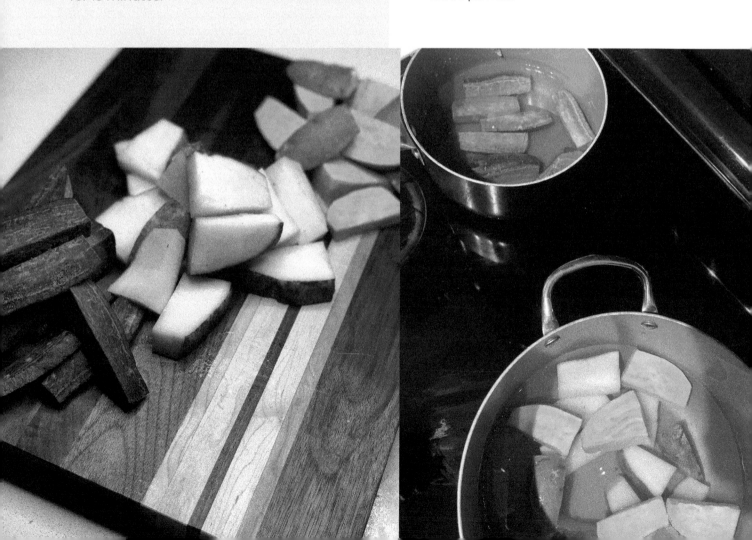

DIRECTIONS

Cut your turnip into fry shaped wedges. Drizzle with a tiny bit of olive oil and make sure the turnip wedges are coated. Sprinkle with salt, pepper and garlic powder. Transfer to air fryer and cook at 375 degrees for 15 minutes checking ½ way and turning.

While they're cooking, chop your tempeh into bite size pieces and warm in a small sauté pan.

When the fries and tempeh are cooked. Place your turnip fries on a large plate and top with tempeh bacon and tomatoes. Drizzle with buffalo sauce and place a heaping tablespoon of vegan sour cream in the center and sprinkle with chopped green onion and cilantro.

Ratings

Calie - These are a weekly staple for me. Fries are literally my favorite food!

Nic – brilliant and so much healthier than getting them from a fast food place!

 9   9

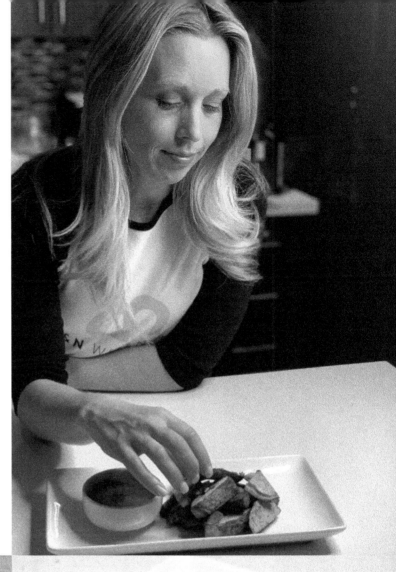

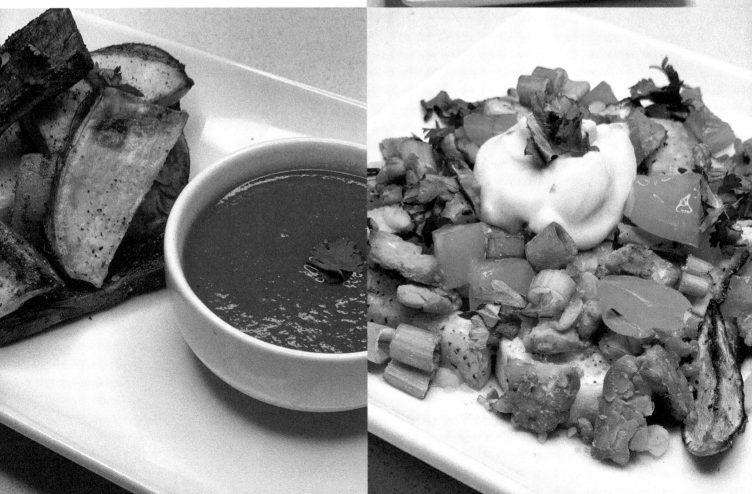

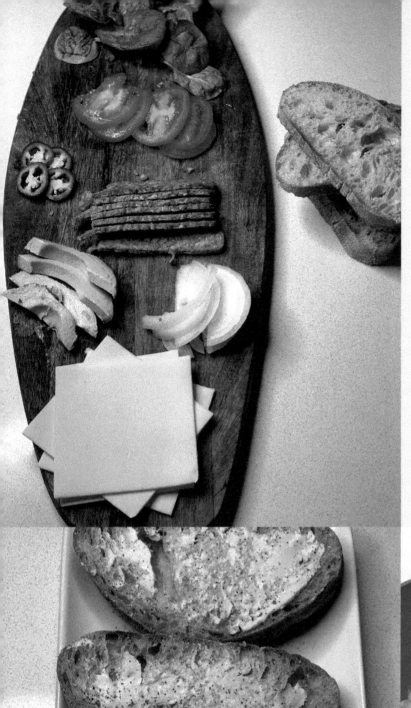

Grown Up BLT

INGREDIENTS

- 2 slices vegan, gluten free bread
- Vegan butter
- Vegan smoked gouda (this makes the dish)
- Smoky tempeh bacon
- Spinach
- Onions
- Tomatoes
- Avocado
- Salt
- Black pepper
- Garlic powder
- Olive oil
- Pickles (optional)
- Jalapeno (optional)

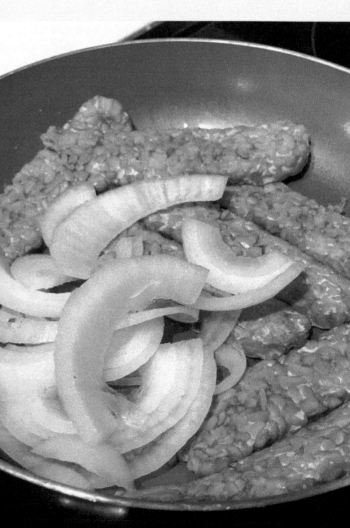

DIRECTIONS

Butter one side of your bread slices and sprinkle with salt, pepper and garlic powder. Set it aside.

In a small sauté pan drizzle a tiny bit of olive oil and add a small handful of sliced onion. Season with a little salt and pepper. Add your smoky tempeh bacon and cook both through. About 5-7 minutes, stirring frequently.

Place your bread butter side down into a sauté pan. Layer your gouda, bacon and onions, spinach, mashed avocado, tomatoes and place your other slice of bread so the butter side is where you can see the butter.

Place a lid on the pan and cook over low heat for about 8 minutes then flip. Place the lid back on your pan and cook an additional 8 minutes until cheese is melted and both sides of the bread are toasted.

Remove from the pan and top with pickle and jalapeno slices. Prepare for your mouth to water!

Ratings

Calie - I wouldn't eat this regularly, but it's the ultimate comfort food to me. Decadent!

10

Nic - no man can miss the meat in this sandwich.

10

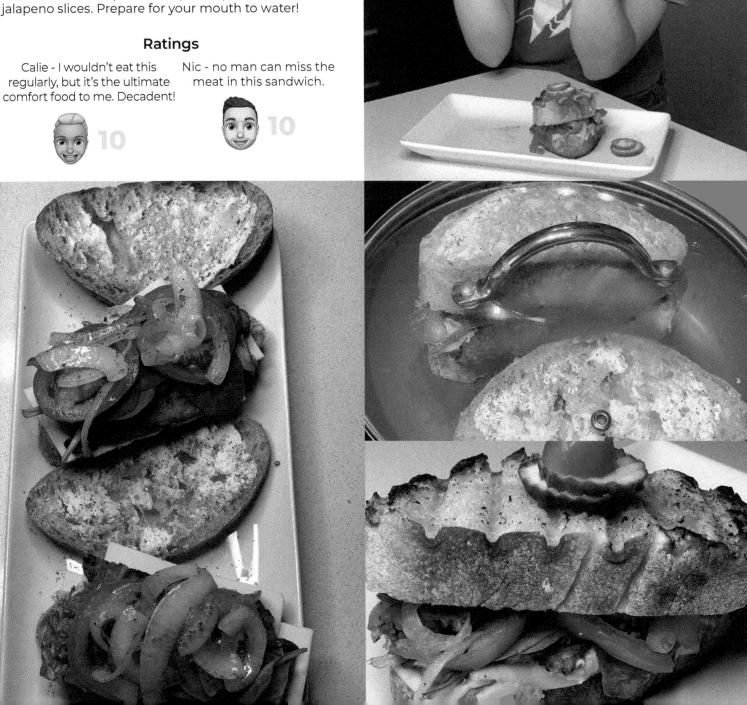

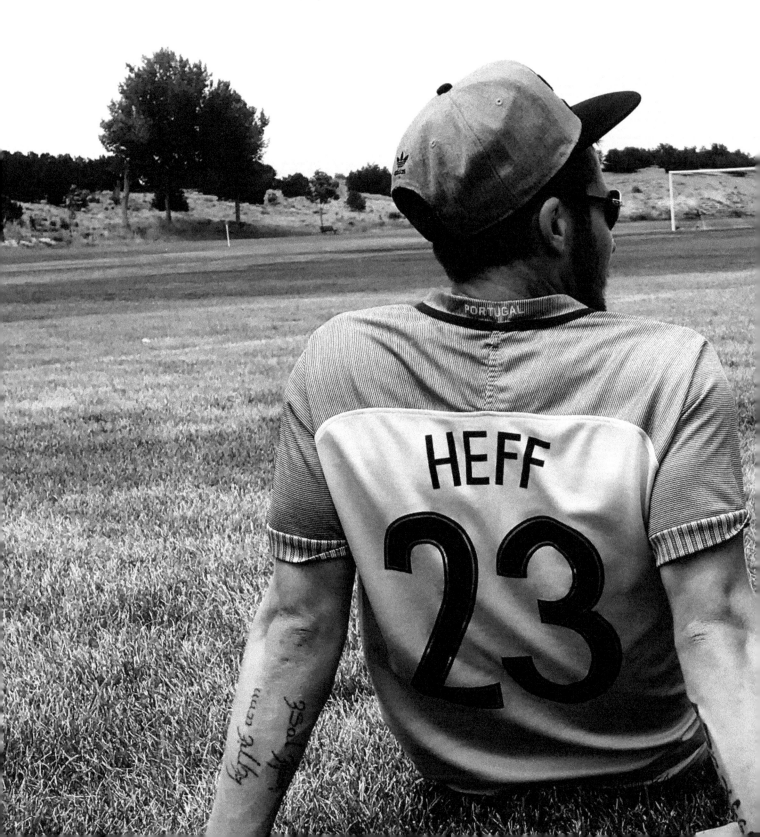

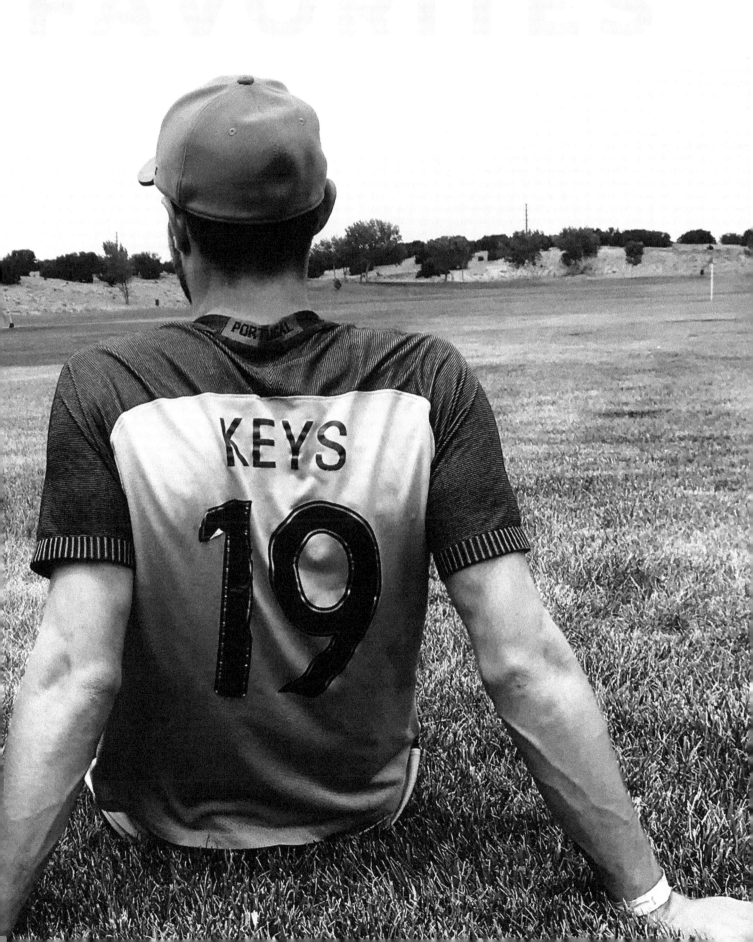

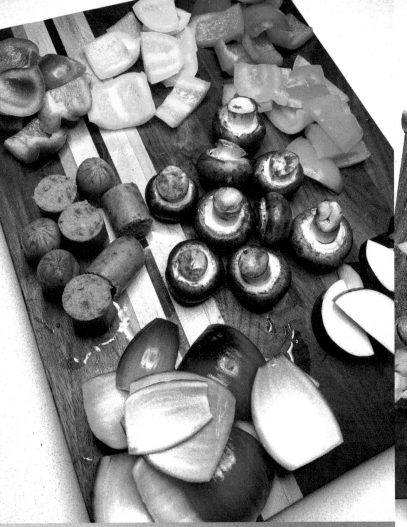

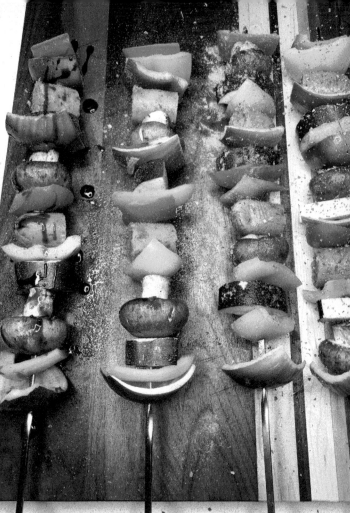

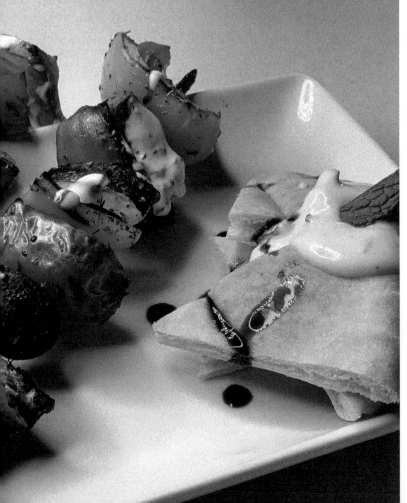

Kebabs

INGREDIENTS

- Veggies of choice (I'm using Red Onion, Peppers, Mushrooms, Zuccini)
- I added Plant-Based Sausage. You can use real meat.
- Olive Oil
- Salt
- Seasonings of choice (I did 2 with curry seasoning and 2 with italian seasoning)
- Balsamic Vinegar (optional)

DIRECTIONS

Preheat Grill or Oven

Cut veggies and plant-based meat if using into thick chunks. Try and make them roughly all the same size so they cook evenly.

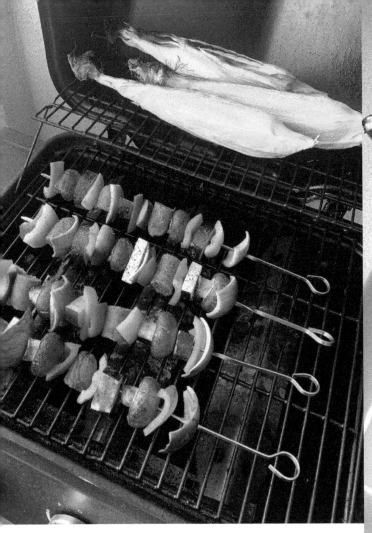

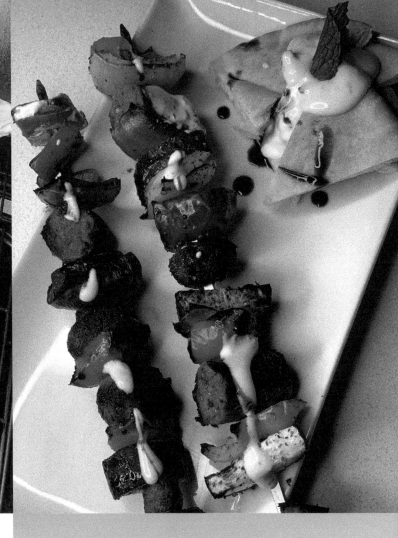

Spray Skewers with Olive Oil spray.

Add veggies chunks to the kebab skewers.

Spray the fully loaded kebabs with oil and then add your seasonings, rotating the kebabs as you go.

Keep rotating every 4 or 5 minutes. Spray them again lightly with oil halfway through cooking.

Once the veggies turn crispy and soft, remove.

Add balsamic vinegar (optional) or a sauce of your choice, and serve.

Ratings

Calie – making these next time I grill with the boys!

 10

Nic – I mean, these are just brilliant

 10

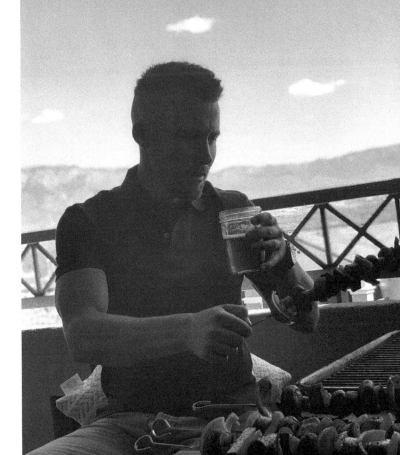

Shepherd's Pie

INGREDIENTS: MASH POTATO TOPPING

- Russet Potatoes or Yukon Gold Potatoes
- 3 tablespoons Olive Oil
- Salt to taste
- 1 Tablespoon of Garlic Powder
- Sour Cream (optional)
- 1 tablespoon of Truffle Oil (optional)

INGREDIENTS: MINCE

- 1 or 2 cups of carrots
- 1 or 2 cups of peas (i use one)
- 1/2 Onion
- 2 cups of Mushrooms
- Plant-Based Ground Meat (Optional, just add 2 more cups of mushrooms if you don't want to use this)
- 4 cloves of garlic
- ¾ cup of chopped Italian Parsley
- Curry Powder (Optional but its my fave for this recipe)
- Gravy (I used Edward & Sons Vegan & Gluten Free Beef Cubes)
- Cheese (optional)

You can honestly add any other veggies to the mince like celery and parsnips.

DIRECTIONS

Cut the potatoes into small pieces. Add into a big pot with around an inch and a half of water. Add some salt. Cover and they should be nice and soft in around 20 mins.

Whilst the potatoes are cooking, start making the mince. In a large pan on medium heat with oil, add the onions, and carrots (and celery/parsnips if using). Sprinkle a little salt and curry powder and cook for around 15 minutes until the carrots are soft and the onions are golden. Now add the mushrooms, peas and garlic. Saute for another 10 minutes. Add the mince and cover on a low heat (I transferred the mix to a medium sized pot as my pan was small).

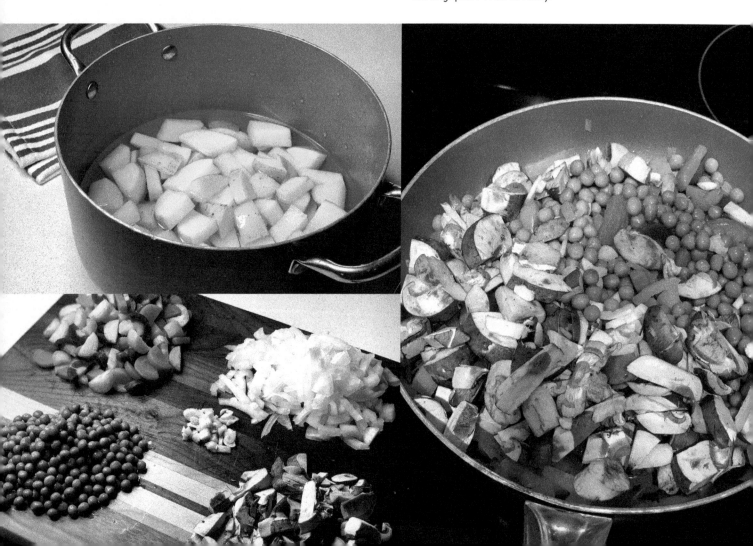

Whilst the mince is cooking, make the gravy (follow instructions on the packet or make your own). Add to the mince pot.

Drain the potatoes and leave in pot. Add 3 tablespoons of olive oil and 1 tablespoon of truffle oil if using. Start mashing! I finish mine off with a scoop of sour cream.

Now stir in your parsley to the mince and fill either a big cooking dish or individual ones like the ones i am using. Top with your mash. To make them look fancy, I cut a whole in the corner of a zip lock bag and used it as a "mashed icing pipe".

Stick them in the oven at 370F for around 20 to 30 minutes until golden brown and bubbly. If adding cheese to the top, sprinkle this on with a few minutes left of cooking time.

Ratings

Calie – really really filling. Well done Nic

 9

Nic - "Reminds me of good ol England"

 10

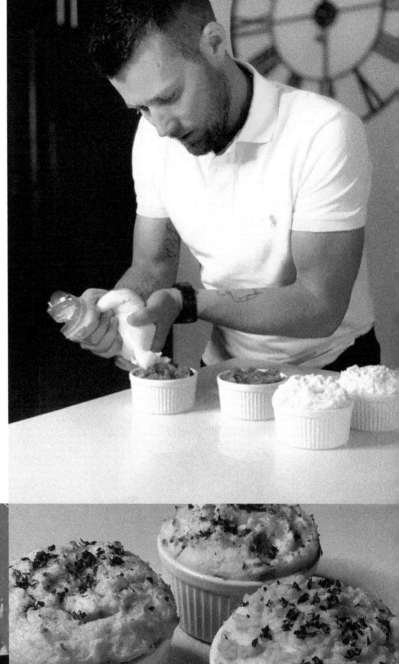

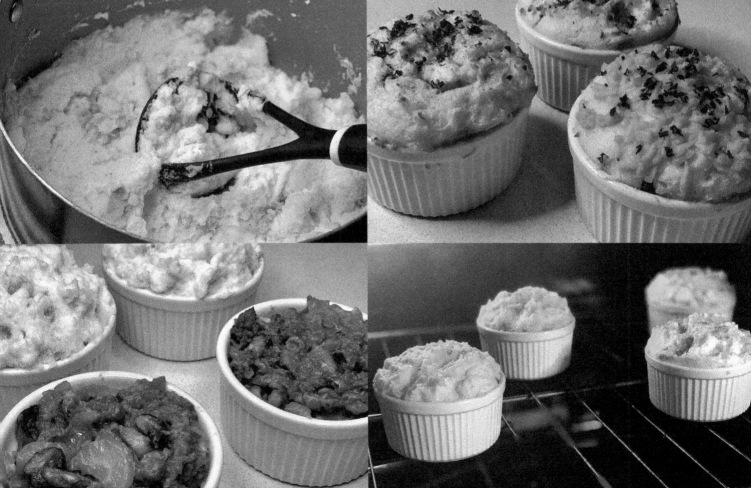

Fish & Chips with Mushy Peas

INGREDIENTS: FISH

- Extra Firm Tofu (one block)
- Sushi Nori Sheets
- Seafood Seasoning
- Garlic Powder
- Salt
- Touch of Pepper

INGREDIENTS: BATTER

- Bottle of Beer (your choice)
- Flour (I used just under 1 cup)
- 2 tsp garlic powder
- 2 salt
- 3 tsp Lemon Juice
- Breadcrumbs

INGREDIENTS: TARTAR SAUCE

- Vegan Mayo
- Gherkins

INGREDIENTS: MUSHY PEAS

- Green Peas
- Lemon Juice
- 1 TBSP Plant-Based Sour Cream
- Oil
- Salt
- Pepper

DIRECTIONS

Before you start, if serving with Fries (I call them chips), and follow those directions accordingly.

Press the tofu (use a store bought press or if you don't have one like me, use a towel). This will get a lot of the moisture out.

Cut the tofu into thick chunks. Make slits on the top of each block, left to right about ½ inch deep. Add a little lemon juice to each tofu piece. Add salt, pepper, garlic and your seafood seasoning in a bowl and mix. Sprinkle on each tofu piece, making sure you season into the slits as well.

In a bowl, mix vegan mayo with chopped gherkins. I also added a little of the gherkin juice as well. Stir. That's your tartar sauce.

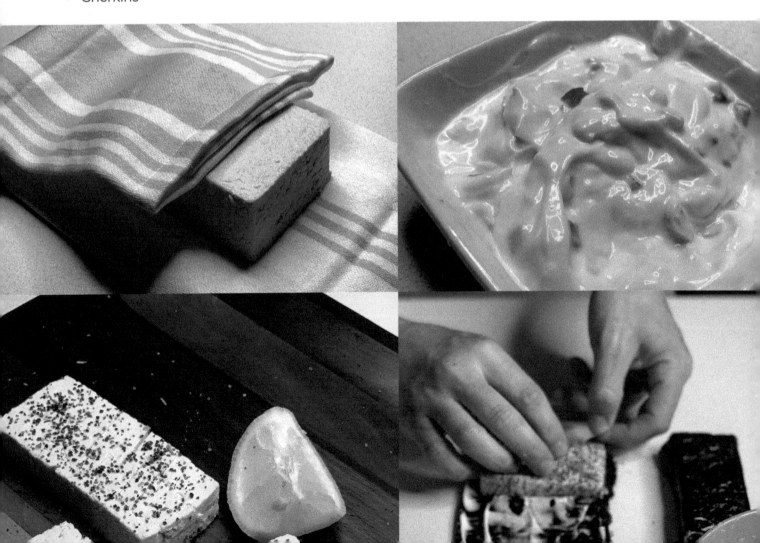

Cut each Sushi Nori Sheet in half. Spread a little of the tartar sauce on each nori sheet with a knife. Grab one of your seasoned tofu pieces and wrap it with the nori sheet. Repeat for the rest.

Mix your beer and seasoning into a bowl. Slowly add flour whilst whisking. Stop when you have your desired batter consistency.

Lay out your breadcrumbs onto a plate. Dunk your tofu pieces into the batter, then roll onto the breadcrumbs, coating the entire tofu piece.

Fry your pieces in hot cooking oil until golden brown (taste better), or use an Air Fryer like I did (healthier).

Whilst the tofu pieces are cooking, mash some peas in a bowl with a little oil, sour cream, lemon juice and salt and pepper to taste.

Serve with fries (chips).

Ratings

Calie – minus those horrible mushy peas

 9

Nic – its really hard to beat real battered fish, but was so surprised with this one!

 8

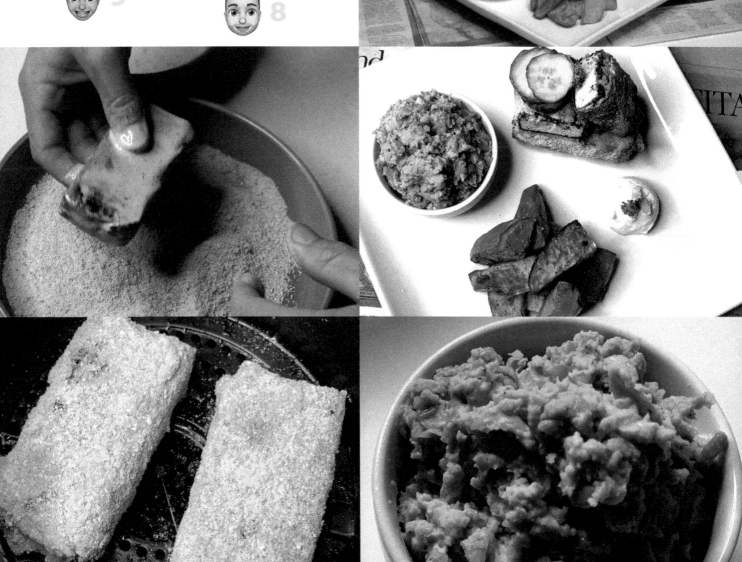